The Hypertension Solution

The Hypertension SOLUTION

Natural Ways to Reverse and Prevent High Blood Pressure

DR. MARK V. WILEY

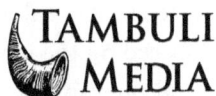

TAMBULI MEDIA

www.TambuliMedia.com

Spring House, PA USA

Revised and Expanded edition of Natural Ways to Reverse and Prevent Hypertension

First Tambuli Media edition, May 08, 2020
www.TambuliMedia.com

ISBN: 978-1-943155-32-3

Library of Congress Control Number: 2020936944

DISCLAIMER

All material in this publication is provided for information only and may not be construed as medical advice. Readers are advised to seek advice from competent medical professionals for their individual health and medical needs. The information and opinions expressed in this publication are believed to be accurate and sound, based on the information available to the author. The editor and publishers are not responsible for errors or omissions.

Contents

Introduction

High Blood Pressure (HBP), medically known as Hypertension, is one of the most prevalent health issues affecting a person's quality of life and longevity. When blood pressure is high undue pressure is placed on artery walls. This forces the heart to pump harder than normal to circulate blood throughout the body. Undiagnosed and/or untreated high blood pressure can put you at risk of heart disease, stroke, kidney disease and other life-threatening diseases—the leading causes of death in the United States.

Statistics offered by the Centers for Disease Control and Prevention (CDCP)[1], paint a scary picture:

- 108 million American adults (45%) have hypertension.

- Less than 24% of Americans have their condition under control.

- 30 million adults diagnosed with high blood pressure do not take their prescribed medication.

- Uncontrolled high blood pressure is common; however, certain groups of people are more

- A greater percent of men (47%) have high blood pressure than women (43%).

- High blood pressure is more common in non-Hispanic black adults (54%) than in non-Hispanic white adults (46%), non-Hispanic Asian adults (39%), or Hispanic adults (36%).

- High blood pressure was a primary or contributing cause of death in 2017 for more than 472,000 people in the United States. That's nearly 1,300 deaths each day.

In addition, The American Heart Association (AHA)[2] reports that:

- 60% of people who have a first heart attack,
- 77% of people who have a first stroke, and
- 74% of people with chronic heart failure have high blood pressure.

What's more, the Mayo Clinic asserts that the cause of high blood pressure is unknown in 85% to 95% of those who have it.[3]

This happens because high blood pressure has a genetic component as well as several external causes. Most people are unknowingly perpetuating multiple causes of their hypertension without even knowing it. The risk factors outlined in this book will give you clear insight into what might be causing your blood pressure to be in a constant elevated state.

High blood pressure is easily diagnosed by using a blood pressure cuff and stethoscope. Your primary care physician can give you the most accurate reading. Conveniently, the machines found in many pharmacies that you insert your arm into to get a blood pressure reading can give you a general idea of your blood pressure condition. Mini blood pressure machines are also now widely available for home use at a reasonable coast from online retailers.

Regardless of whether you already suffer from hypertension, prevention is the best defense. Happily, the means of reversing hypertension and the means of preventing it are one and the same: That is, understanding its cause and adopting the necessary and simple lifestyle changes.

While prescription medications can effectively reduce your blood pressure, and are effective at saving lives, they do not address the root causes of hypertension. As such, if you follow this therapy and make no other changes in your life, you will forever have to rely on prescription medication to keep your blood pressure under control. And once you stop taking the drugs, your blood pressure will again rise. Please take hold of your situation and make the necessary lifestyle changes required to reverse and prevent this potentially life-threatening condition.

The Hypertension Solution offers real strategies you can embrace to eradicate from your life the ill-effects of unresolved high blood pressure. It offers a clear-cut and comprehensive approach steeped in natural supplementation, dietary changes, stress reduction techniques, safe exercises and simple mind-body practices like yoga and meditation.

Taken as a whole, the information presented herein is really a case for modifying your lifestyle and making healthy choices that keep blood pressure within the normal, healthy range. The rest of your life begins now, why not begin the wellness process today? You can, and I believe in you.

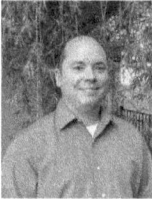

Yours in Optimal Health,

MARK WILEY, OMD, PhD, MS
Self-Directed Wellness Advocate

CHAPTER 1

Hypertension and its Risk Factors

High blood pressure (HBP) is at epidemic proportions among Americans. Luckily, there are easy and natural ways to reduce, control and prevent hypertension. Before we get into them, it is best to have at least a cursory understanding of the disease and its risk factors.

WHAT IS HYPERTENSION?

Blood pressure is a measurement reading of the amount of force the heart generates while pumping blood through the arteries. There are two numbers involved in the reading of blood pressure: Systolic and diastolic. Systolic represents the amount of force expended by the heart as it fills the blood vessels. Diastolic pressure, on the other hand, is a numeric quantification of the resistance to that force. When taken together, the systolic and diastolic numbers provide an indication of how successful your heart is at getting the blood to the tissues in your body.

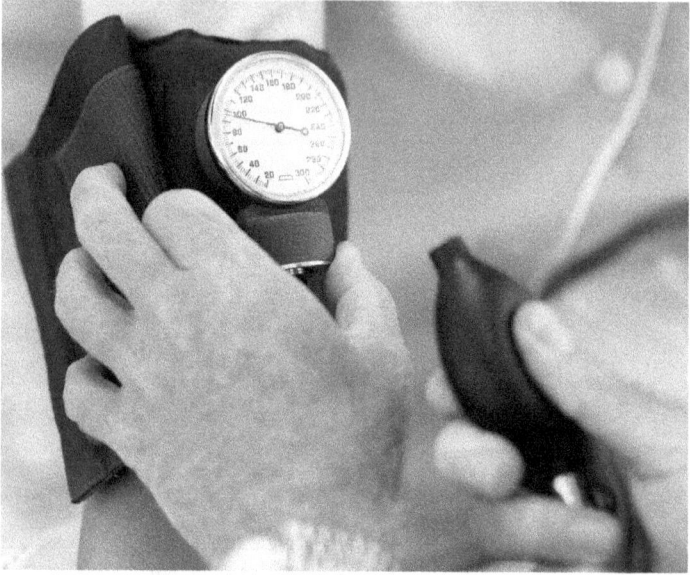

The medically healthy range is a reading below 120 (systolic) and 80 (diastolic) pressure, commonly represented as 120/80 mmHg. Hypertension is clinically defined as a blood pressure reading above 140/90 mmHg. Left unchecked, HBP can lead to very serious health issues, including stroke, heart disease, arterial aneurysms, hardening of the arteries and kidney failure.

There are two types of hypertension to be aware of. When no specific cause of contracting this health issue is identified, it is known as *essential hypertension*. Hypertension that is caused by a pre-existing health condition (e.g., stress, adrenal gland tumor, arteriosclerosis, diabetes, obesity, kidney disease), the side effect of medication (e.g., birth control pills, some cold remedies, corticosteroids, migraine meds), or from poor lifestyle choices (e.g., alcohol abuse, high salt intake) is termed *secondary hypertension.*

ELUSIVE SIGNS AND SYMPTOMS

The scariest thing about hypertension is that it can kill without showing specific signs of being present. In other words, *there are no signs and symptoms of poor health that are specific to the identification of hypertension.* You see, while its symptoms include headache, blurry vision and dizziness, these are not specific to high blood pressure alone, and can be present for any number of related or unrelated reasons. That is why hypertension is called, "the silent killer."

As a result of its lack of specific symptoms, hypertension is often detected too late—that is, when one's blood pressure is far above healthy limits and within a potentially lethal range. When blood pressure is in this range, some combination of the following symptoms will be present: Severe headache, fatigue or confusion, chest pain, difficulty breathing, irregular heartbeat, blood in the urine and pounding in your chest, neck or ears.[4]

If you are experiencing any of the above-mentioned symptoms, see your physician immediately. It's possible that you may be experiencing what is known as a "hypertensive crisis." If this is the case, it can lead to stroke or heart attack and can result in heart, brain and kidney damage.[5]

Hypertension is difficult to diagnose without taking your blood pressure on a regular basis. What's more, it does not discriminate in who it affects. Getting a handle on early warning signs by knowing the risk factors and your relationship with them, is a big step toward prevention.

By knowing what your individual risks are you can keep an eye on things and take the necessary steps to reverse or prevent hypertension, thereby reducing your chances of experiencing hypertension-related heart attack, heart disease or stroke. Below are the most common risk factors by category that are associated with hypertension.

Genetics—High blood pressure has a genetic component, so people whose parents, siblings or close relatives have (or have had) hypertension are at increased risk of developing it.

Ethnicity—African Americans and Native- Americans are more likely candidates to develop hypertension than are Caucasian-Americans and Mexican- Americans. They also are predisposed to developing it earlier in life.[6]

Gender—Men are also more likely to develop hypertension at an earlier age than women. In fact, high blood pressure affects significantly more men under age 45 than women in the same age group. Beginning at age 65, women are at higher risk than men for developing high blood pressure because their blood vessels become less flexible.

In addition to the areas listed above for which we have *no* control over, lifestyle choices play a major role in the development of hypertension over the course of one's life. And this we *do* have control over. This means that we have the ability, through our actions and choices, to cause, reverse and prevent this potentially life-threatening condition. Here's what you need to know:

Poor Health—The onset of secondary hypertension can be caused by other ill-health conditions such as those associated with the kidneys, adrenals and arteries. And diseases affecting these are often caused by poor diet, lack of exercise and stress. In other words, they are preventable and thus self-induced by poor lifestyle choices.

Excess Weight—Obese and overweight people are at high risk of hypertension. It has repeatedly been shown that losing weight can lower your blood pressure by about 5 mm/Hg per 10 pounds of weight loss. People who have a body mass index (BMI) of 25 or greater are more likely to have high blood pressure than people who weigh less. Here is a website where you can calculate your BMI: http://www.bmi-calculator.net

High Sodium Intake—The consumption of too much salt puts you at risk for developing hypertension. Your kidneys simply can't process excessive salt consumption. Reduce your salt and your blood pressure will also reduce.

Alcohol Consumption—Studies show that consuming more than three alcoholic beverages per day will dramatically raise your blood pressure. Cut back and your blood pressure goes down.

Smoking—You place yourself at risk every time you inhale a cancer stick, I mean cigarette. Smoking temporarily elevates blood pressure by 5 mm/Hg to 10 mm/Hg for about a half-hour. If you smoke a pack a day and already have high blood pressure, you are exponentially increasing your risk of death.

Poor Diet—A diet high in calories, fat and sugar can cause weight gain and the development of hypertension. Moreover, deficiency in vitamin D in women and a high consumption of fructose and high fructose corn syrup have also been associated with an elevated risk of hypertension.

Physical Inactivity—A sedentary lifestyle and a general lack of daily exercise increases not only your risk of hypertension, but also your risk of developing obesity and heart disease. Regular exercise helps to control blood pressure, thus making it one of the best options for preventing and curing this disease.

Stress—Studies have shown that people with heightened anxiety, intense anger and suppressed expression of anger are more at risk of developing high blood pressure.[7]

PRESCRIPTION MEDICATIONS

The pharmaceutical companies have developed some fine drugs for treating hypertension. These include diuretics, angiotensin converting enzymes, angiotensin receptor blockers, alpha blockers, beta blockers, calcium channel blockers and vasodilators.[8] These pharmaceuticals respectively increase the elimination of sodium, inhibit the hormones that cause blood pressure to rise, alter the involuntary nervous system to force a decrease in pressure, reduce blood vessel constriction and dilate arteries to decrease overall pressure.

The problem is that prescription drug therapy is often used too late; that is, after the diagnosis of hypertension has been given. Often, the prescriptions must be taken in combination and they must be taken for the remainder of one's life. While drugs can remove the symptoms and side effects of hypertension during the time they are being taken, they do not reverse or prevent high blood pressure from developing. Therefore, they should be thought of as a temporary first line to help reduce symptoms while you get your lifestyle changes in place.

THE NATURAL APPROACH

The best way to avoid the health risks of hypertension is simply to prevent it from occurring in the first place. With regular monitoring of your blood pressure readings as confirmation of the positive changes you will make toward lowering stress, eating more healthfully, increasing daily exercise and realigning lifestyle choices, reversal of the disease and prevention of its return will not be far behind. The following sections of this book will show you how.

Lowering your systolic blood pressure by 2 mm/Hg, you can reduce your risk of dying from heart disease by 7% and of dying from a stroke by 10%.

Simple changes to lifestyle can reduce blood pressure naturally and without medication. Stress is also a major culprit in the blood pressure battle. Stress causes bodily tension, restricted breathing and rising of blood pressure. If you feel stressed out frequently or have a stressful job, engaging in daily mind/body practices like yoga and meditation has been shown to reduce hypertension. Diet is another important first line of defense. For some, this is as easy as cutting out potato chips, not salting foods and limiting canned and processed meats, especially cold cuts. Overall, there are five areas that you can modify in your life, each effecting positive change to your health and lowering blood pressure. These are: reducing stress, engaging in safe exercise, changing your diet, taking supplements or Chinese herbals, and receiving energy-work therapy. Each of these areas are discusses in detail in the chapters that follow.

CHAPTER 2

The Stress, High Blood Pressure Connection

Stress is one of the leading causes of illness in the United States. Nearly 66% of all signs and symptoms presented in doctors' offices in the United States are either cause by stress or related to its side effects.

The negative effects include nail biting, anxiety, a racing mind, obsessive thoughts, compulsive behavior, unending worry, muscle tension and spasm, poor appetite or too great an appetite, digestive disorders, constipation, insomnia, poor blood flow, belabored breathing, neck pain, shoulder tension and the possible onset or continuation of bad habits like alcohol dependence, drug use, abuse of pain killers and the over consumption of food and caffeine.

Stress is a normal and necessary process for our survival. However, too much stress, a combination of mental, physical, emotional, chemical or environmental stress, and stress left unresolved over extended periods of time, can lead to serious health problems like high blood pressure, heart disease and stroke. Natural and simple ways of reducing stress, without a doubt, are essential to any therapeutic hypertension program.

THE PSYCHOLOGY OF STRESS

Stress is an interesting phenomenon and it means different things to different people. What we each individually consider to be stressful is largely a matter of our perception. Indeed, our perceptions form and inform our realities and so what we think is posing a threat is doing so by virtue of our established belief system. Moreover, there are many kinds of stressors—physical (e.g., the response to being frightened), emotional (e.g., loss of a loved one), psychological (e.g., obsessive thoughts), spiritual (e.g., loss of faith) and psychosomatic (e.g., the need for attention).

Physiologically, stress is responsible for initiating the fight or flight response in the face of perceived danger. This means that when we are confronted with a danger, our body automatically prepares us to deal with the coming stressful situation by focusing our attention, pumping more blood into our muscles and sending the stress hormones adrenaline and cortisol through our system. It is precisely this response that helps protect the body and return it again to homeostasis (our balanced, baseline of wellness).

However, at the conclusion of the danger episode the body does not as automatically calm down and return to homeostasis (its

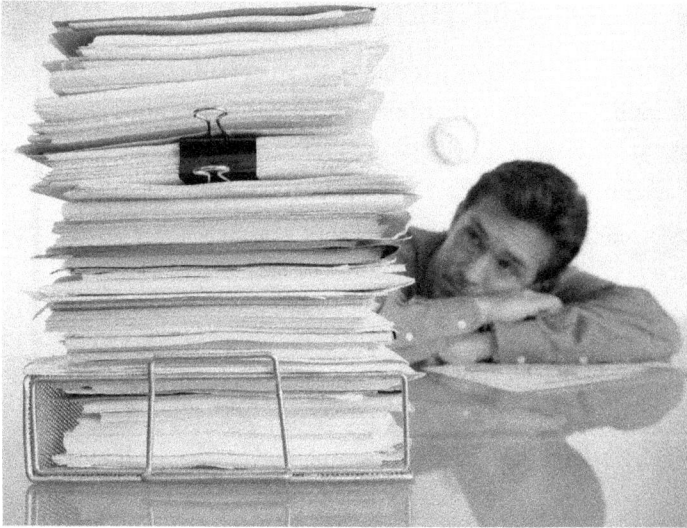

natural balanced state). In fact, it takes a great deal of time for the body to return to so-called normal conditions. But often this cannot happen because another stressor may present itself (e.g., sitting in traffic, standing in line at the bank, missing a deadline) and this will send our body into "code red" mode all over again.

Our inability to deal with stress creates severe biochemical imbalances in our body and prevents it from reestablishing homeostasis. Therefore, without learning to come to terms with our perceptions that cause the stress that leads to physiological, psychological, physical and emotional triggers that cause pain, illness and disease, we can never truly become "well." One of the key elements of this state is raised blood pressure.

Stressful episodes of nervousness, worry, anger or physically demanding work temporarily raise blood pressure. When the stressor or stressful situation is removed, blood pressure goes back down. When the stressful event occurs again, blood pressure again rises. The problem occurs when stress is maintained at a high level for an extended period.

Hypertension research scientists are unsure at this point about the possible effects of long-term stress on high blood pressure. They believe that long-term stress can contribute to hypertension, but they are not sure how much of an impact it may have. In the case of short-term stressful situations, they know that stress can make blood pressure go up for a while. But once the stressor is removed or the situation is resolved, blood pressure readings return to normal. However, the removal and relief of stress is not always possible, thereby extending the duration of the raise in blood pressure. This is harmful because even

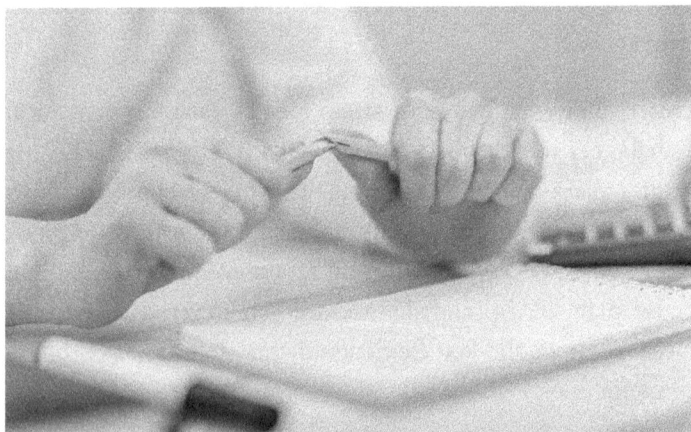

if you do not actually have hypertension, the body is held in a pattern mimicking the ill effects of the disease. And if the effects are there long enough, you can then be said to have developed the disease. Getting a handle on stress is the way to avoid this. But how can you know when you've reached your normal coping capacity and have allowed your stress to move into dangerous territory?

Your body's display of signs and symptoms is its natural means of communicating that something is wrong. It is way out of balance. Many people ignore the warning signs of stress. They think it is normal to feel exhausted, "burned out," unable to concentrate and to drink or eat too much to deal with anxiety--induced from their stressful situation. This is not normal, but it has become the way of life for millions of Americans. Working through the symptoms, dealing with the problems, pushing ahead and proving to yourself, taking over the counter (OTC) or prescription pills to stay level... everyone is doing it! But these signs are telling you to slow down. If not, you may be headed for serious health problems. There are warning signs of stress you need to pay attention to. The box below lists the physical, mental, emotional and behavioral signs and symptoms that are related to stress and may also be indicators of hypertension.[9]

Physical Signs—Dizziness, general aches and pains, grinding teeth, clenched jaws, headaches, indigestion, muscle tension, difficulty sleeping, racing heart, ringing in the ears, stooped posture, sweaty palms, tiredness, exhaustion, trembling, weight gain or loss, upset stomach

Mental Signs—Constant worry, difficulty making decisions, forgetfulness, inability to concentrate, lack of creativity, loss of sense of humor

Emotional Signs—Anger, anxiety, crying, depression, feeling powerless, frequent mood swings, irritability, loneliness, negative thinking, nervousness, sadness

Behavioral Signs—Bossiness, compulsive eating, critical attitude of others, explosive actions, frequent job changes, impulsive actions, increased use of alcohol or drugs, withdrawal from relationships or social situations

THE STRESS CYCLE

The vicious cause-and-effect cycle associated with stress is readily seen in our workplace where the pressure of productivity and the meeting of deadlines and bottom-line expectations lead us down a harrowing path. Consider the average day in the life of a corporate worker: Wakes up early, skips breakfast and rushes to the office; begins harboring stress and anxiety while watching the clock sitting in traffic; sits all days at the computer and/or negotiates personalities on the phone; takes breaks, not to stretch and take deep breaths of fresh air, but to artificially stimulate the body to work harder by puffing on cigarettes and downing another cup of coffee; then it's back to work, pushing himself in an attempt to meet expectations wherein stress and tensions rise and take hold of the body. After work, to relax, office co-workers are joined for happy hour, and the body is nourished with more caffeine, cigarettes, fast food and too much alcohol. Later that evening the body and mind are wound so tight and so stressed that there is no way to achieve deep, restful sleep.

Round and round, day after day it goes until the body finally rebels and "tells" you something is very wrong by way of an ulcer, gastrointestinal disorder or chronic pain in some manifestation. Years later, your doctor diagnoses your nagging symptoms as hypertension. Knowing the risks and poor lifestyle choices that over time cause high blood pressure, this should come as no surprise. Getting enough deep sleep is one of the easiest and most natural ways the body can repair the negative effects of daily stress and re-balance its blood pressure. Unfortunately for many, a full night's sleep is a dream they once had.

SLEEP YOUR STRESS AWAY

Not only is sleep a fundamental human need, it is a necessity that no one who experiences poor health of any kind should ever take for granted. It is so important, in fact, that we naturally fall asleep when our bodies tell our brains that certain essential chemicals have been depleted and our muscles and organs are tired and in need of restoration.

The growing problem is that many of us rely on legal stimulants like coffee, tea, soda and energy drinks to force ourselves to remain awake and continue plugging away.

Work, after all, can't be held back by pleading with the boss or client. There just are not enough hours in the week. The result? We stay up too late and we get up too early and, to do this, we consume unhealthy amounts of toxic substances—day after night after day.

The net result is poor concentration, slower reaction times, decreased performance levels, less ability to learn and compartmentalize new skills and knowledge, more frequent memory lapses, increases in simple injuries and accidents, adverse changes in moods and behaviors and an increased frequency of headaches, neck and shoulder pain, backaches, fatigue and overload of toxic beverage consumption. These all can lead to high blood pressure.

During sleep, the body is working to repair itself. The liver purifies blood, the muscles repair and serotonin increases. Without ample sleep, these things do not happen at optimal levels. In our natural circadian rhythm—or biological clock—sleep is set to take over during the evening hours. We are genetically programmed to get up and lie down with the sun. It was the invention of artificial sources of light (candles and then light bulbs) that began our stressed-out drive for more working hours at the expense of much-needed rest.

What's the big deal, you ask, if you sleep only a few hours per night? You can always drink coffee, consume energy drinks, take caffeine pills or snatch a cat nap. Well, not really. Did you know that in clinical tests rats die within a few short weeks of sleep deprivation? And it's not just rats at risk. Harvard Medical School researchers correlated the association between lack of sleep and hypertension, heart attack and cancer.[10]

Chronic fatigue, adrenal fatigue, attention deficit disorder, chronic migraine and headache, body aches and pain, mental illness, depression and anxiety are all in part caused—or made worse—by lack of sleep. It is essential for those with episodic high blood pressure or full-blown hypertension to do their best to get eight hours of sound, restful sleep per night.

7 SLEEP TIPS FOR RESTFUL SLEEP

1) Do not consume ANY sugar or caffeine after 6:00 pm.

2) Stop working at least two hours before bedtime.

3) Turn off the computer and television at least one hour before bedtime.

4) Make sure your sleeping quarters are as dark and silent as possible. Studies have shown that those in darker and quieter spaces tend to sleep through the night more deeply than others.

5) Establish a sleep/wake schedule and stick to it.

6) Make a set routine out of bedtime. Change into pajamas, brush your teeth, set out clothes for the morning, even jot down any last thoughts but promise yourself to revisit them tomorrow, then turn off the light... breathe deep, relax, sleep tight.

7) If your racing mind is nagging, meditate. (Described in the next chapter.)

There are several techniques for helping one do this. Below are Seven Tips to help decrease the frequency and duration of insomnia to help you get your eight hours of restful sleep.

For those who exercise at night... flip your schedule!

It's keeping you up by moving blood and energy through your system. Researchers at Stanford University School of Medicine found that adults ages 55 to 75 who engaged in 20-to-30 minutes of low-impact exercise (like walking) every other day in the afternoon, were able to fall asleep in half their normal time. What's more, their sleep duration increased on average by one full hour![11]

What does all this mean? Good health begins as easily and naturally as putting in plenty of sack time. Try for a straight eight hours. And maybe think about buying a new set of sheets to celebrate the new healthier happier sounder sleeping you!

The idea behind living a stress-free life is to remove the things in your life that are causing you to be stressed. Of course, this is easier said than done, but it is truly the only way not to have stress. For most people, this is impossible, as their relationship with work, their financial situation and the people around them create their stress. Mind-body techniques for "reframing" the way those things are perceived are described in Chapter 3. For now, here are 10 simple things you can do daily to reduce the symptoms of stress.

A good stress-relief program should be sought and followed. Good programs generally include various forms of meditation, visualization, qigong, yoga, acupressure and biofeedback. Not all programs contain everything but engaging in any or some of these will go a long way to reclaiming years for your life. The following chapters discuss these methods in more detail.

10 STRESS BUSTERS

1) Walk outside for at least 20 continuous minutes every day.

2) Take the stairs whenever possible.

3) Take 10 deep belly breaths every hour.

4) Drink plenty of pure water—at least 10 glasses a day.

5) Avoid sugar and caffeine in all forms.

6) Regulate sleep and wake cycles to a consistent daily routine.

7) Prioritize your life, work, family and personal time and activities.

8) Do six shoulder shrugs whenever you are tense.

9) Realize that when people criticize and judge, they are labeling an "image" of you and not you personally.

10) Realize that you are worth so much more than the sum of your titles, money and belongings.

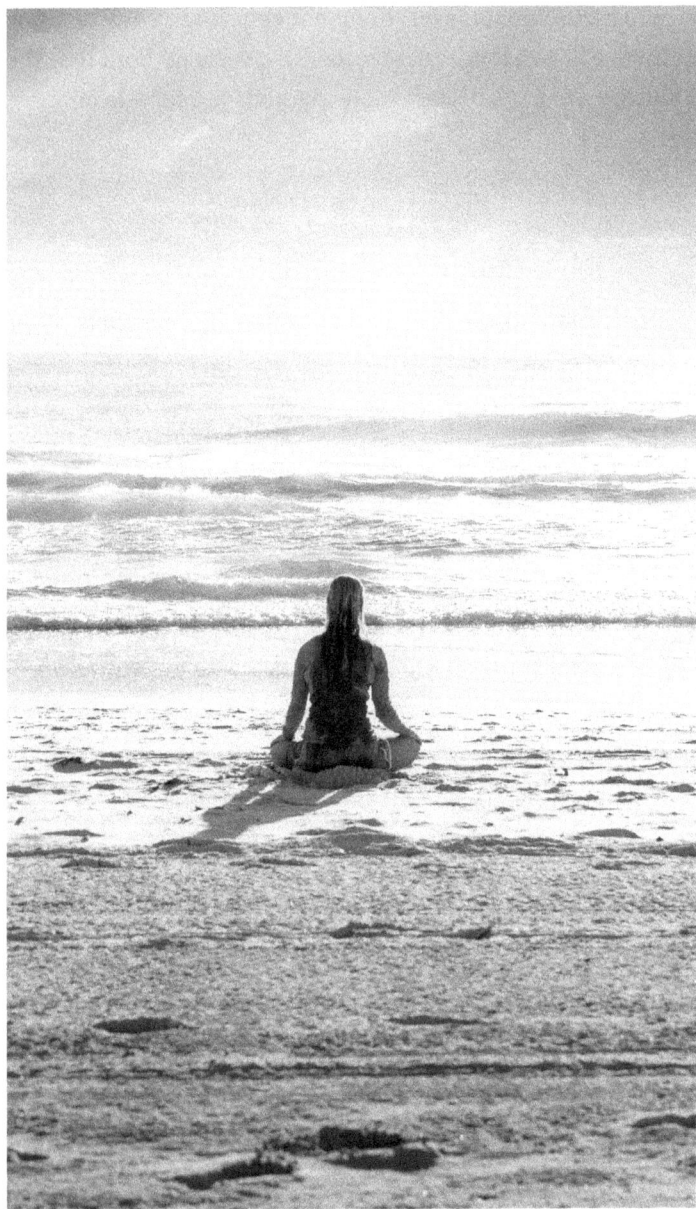

CHAPTER 3

Mind–Body Practices for Reducing Stress and Blood Pressure

There are many causes of stress, high blood pressure and ill health. Yet despite high-tech medical advances, low-tech massage and other treatments, people are still suffering. The answer may well be found within the mind and the hold it has over our thoughts, emotions and our physical bodies. When the mind (psycho) and the body (soma) come together in adverse ways to manifest, aggravate or prolong episodes of stress and elevated blood pressure, you are at risk of serious and potentially life-threatening health issues like heart disease and stroke.

MIND-BODY MEDICINE

In decades past, the term psychosomatic was primarily used by psychologists to identify pains or illnesses that were "all in the mind" and "not real." This outlook is markedly outdated and false. The mind is so powerful it has within itself the ability to heal the body. Practices like yoga, qigong and meditation were once considered the esoteric domain of traditional cultures. Today in the West, however, they are now considered mainstream practices and fall under the wellness classification known as "mind-body medicine."

The practices of mind-body medicine include those techniques that help create an environment where in the mind can affect the function and symptoms of the body. These methods include deep breathing, meditation, visualization, slow movements and exercises, prayer, chanting and listening to soothing sounds and music. Mind-body medicine also incorporates various psychological techniques for clearing out old, harmful thought patterns and the way in which events are perceived.

In the following sections we will look at the mind-body practices like The Sedona Method™, Neuro-Linguistic Programming, and several methods of Meditation, Qigong and Yoga.

THE SEDONA METHOD™

Pioneered by Lester Levenson, The Sedona Method™ is a powerful yet easy-to-learn technique that teaches you how to "let go" of unwanted emotions in an instant. When left unresolved, negative emotions can cause symptoms of ill-health—symptoms that include stress, pain, anxiety and high blood pressure. Essentially, The Sedona Method™ consists of a series of questions you ask yourself that leads your awareness to what you are feeling in the moment and then gently guides you into the experience of letting go.

This method is easy to do because there are only a few steps necessary to accomplish the release of new or decades-old pent up negative emotions. With so many successes, this again points to the vital role the mind and emotions play in the health issues we suffer in our bodies—those psychosomatic illnesses.

The effectiveness of The Sedona Method™ has been validated by respected scientific researchers at major universities and by the MONY Corporation. In fact, practitioners of this method tell us that if you're not feeling happy, confident and relaxed at least 90% of the time, then chances are manifestations of ill health are tied to unresolved negative emotions.

The Sedona Method's™ "releasing" operates on the "feeling" level make it an easy process. It teaches you to "let go" of years of mental programs and accumulated feelings in just seconds.

There is a comprehensive book on this method available everywhere, titled The Sedona Method™,[12] and tons of free videos are available online. Please look and see how this mind-body method might help you resolve unwanted emotional toxicity from your life to reduce your stress and lower your blood pressure.

NEURO-LINGUISTIC PROGRAMMING (NLP)

Neuro-Linguistic Programming (NLP) is the art of under-standing and communicating with our minds. It breaks down this way: Neuro (understanding the nervous system and the five senses), linguistic (understanding language and how it really affects our minds), and programming (understanding our ability to organize our neurological systems—thought processes).

In terms of biological warning signs like elevated blood pressure, headache, blurry vision and the inability to focus or get sound sleep, it is important to keep in mind that many adverse health symptoms are merely "information" provided by your body. When there is a problem with your body, it communicates this to your brain via nerve impulses. These impulses are "signals" that send the symptomatic information to the brain to make you uncomfortable to force you to do something about it and return the body to its balanced state.

NLP teaches you is to take control of your thoughts and how to become free to change your mind… about what you are thinking and how you are thinking about it. If you understand the way your brain processes information and you understand why and how language impacts your feelings, then you will start to see you can reprogram your mind and change the way you feel. And the way you feel is generally a response to and an indicator of the quality of your health.

NLP can be used in many ways and for many things. One way is through a technique known as "reframing." Reframing is a nice way to start using basic NLP principles. It's easy and it shows you that your outlook on life has a lot to do with the life you lead. Reframing is your first step toward a more positive mindset regarding stress and hypertension and for your whole life.

Let's think about the symptoms of stress and hypertension for a moment. These include: Headache, fatigue, confusion, anxiety, insomnia, chest pain, difficulty breathing, irregular heartbeat and more. As stated earlier, adverse health symptoms are simply a form of communication. You may say to yourself, "My head hurts, I am feeling anxious, I need more sleep, my blood pressure is high and I need to see my doctor because I am afraid I may have a serious health problem."

According to practitioners of NLP, what you in fact are doing by stating this concern (which you might do repeatedly to as many people as will listen) is letting yourself know you have all these problems. By focusing on the problems, you are re-affirming a negative cycle. The practice of NLP can "reframe" the above negative thought pattern into a positive one.

"Stress is killing me with all these symptoms. My body is telling me to be careful and slow down before my episodic high blood pressure becomes full-blown hypertension. Ok, I should do some mind-body exercises and be sure to get enough sleep to release these symptoms. I must also be aware that I need to watch out for things that could add too much pressure to my life at this point. I am vulnerable and it is good that my body reminds me through these symptoms to look after my health. So, to thank my body I must keep up with my natural program of reversing and preventing hypertension."

Rather than fighting against the information—fighting the message—you can use reframing to acknowledge the problem and take affirmative action steps to reduce and eliminate your elevated stress and blood pressure. Then, while engaged in your corrective program, you will be mindful to listen to the communication of information from your body to your brain and acknowledge the relief as it comes... slow or fast.

Here are the basic steps:

1) Identify the problem
2) Separate the intention from the learned behavior
3) Set a positive way forward.

Identifying the problem sounds easy, but often we react rather than reason. So, the first thing to do is take a moment to be with your symptoms and assess them so you can understand the why, when and how of them. Why is it happening (e.g., your diet is poor, and you smoke)? When is it happening (e.g., during stressful periods of work or family time)? What is happening (e.g., pounding headaches, chest pain, insomnia)? How is it happening (e.g., it is fear-based as you worry that it will get bad, so you get in the mindset of being in pain)?

To separate the intention from the learned behavior, you must slow down to really talk to yourself about a better way to deal with the problem at hand. You might say, "Okay, I know I am having negative symptoms related to stress and high blood pressure, but it's not a disease and it's reversible and preventable." Thinking and acknowledging in this way keeps you focused on getting to step three.

To set a positive way forward, you can thank your body for the message of pain, as it focused you to work with better intention for achieving your best health and long- term life goals. You can reframe in many ways, just look at the positive view of the situation and let your mind work for you!

MEDITATION'S TRANSFORMATIVE NATURE

Meditation is practiced in countless ways. Each country and each religion have its own means of meditation for spiritual discipline, healing practice or mechanism for psychological growth. People engage in meditation because they find it empowering, rewarding, healing, meaningful, peaceful... and much more. For those under constant stress and suffering hypertension, it can be transforming.

Meditation is one of the great boons to personal health and well-being. When people meditate, they come to terms with

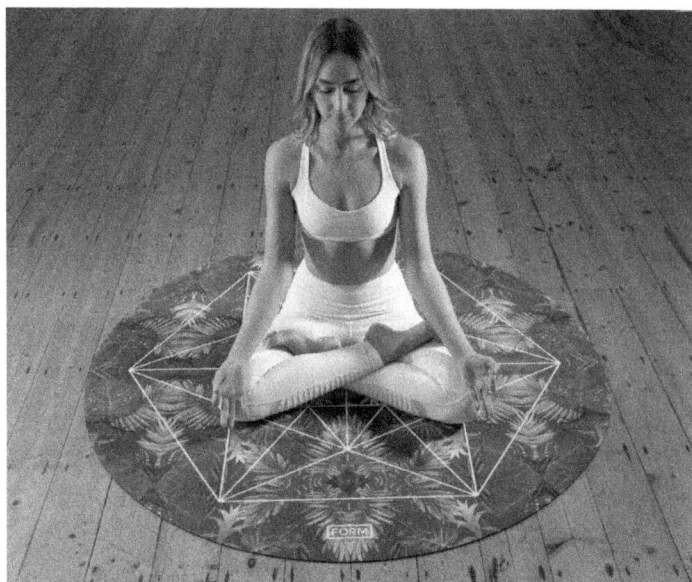

themselves, alone, free from the overt distractions of the outside world. It is through the act and process of meditation that you can examine your health, your pain, your symptoms, your mind, yourself. I am a big fan of meditation; I suggest you try it, too. There are many different meditation techniques and methods out there but choosing the right one for you need not be a daunting process. All you need is a brief introduction to get you started.

Meditation is practiced in countless ways. Each country and religion have its own means of meditating for spiritual discipline or healing practice or as a mechanism for psychological growth. People engage in meditation because they find it empowering, rewarding, healing, meaningful, peaceful… and so much more. For those under constant stress and suffering from conditions like hypertension, anxiety, depression, insomnia and pain, meditation can be transforming.

ZAZEN MEDITATION—Zazen or seated Zen meditation is a Japanese practice that derives from Buddhism. It is a philosophy or a way of life, thinking and being. Its goal is to bring your mind into the present moment and to hold a single point of focus or attention. The meditative aspect of Zen uses phrases known as koans, which are non-logical or nonsensical. A familiar example is, "What is the sound of one hand clapping?" The purpose of repeating a phrase that makes no sense or cannot be solved is to occupy your mind for long periods of time without it drifting from the task. In other words, you reduce the risk of mental distraction during the practice of meditation.

Here are the basic steps:

1) Sit in a relaxed position with the spine straight. Many practitioners choose to sit on a cushion that elevates them slightly, helps hold their spine erect and makes sitting for long periods more comfortably.

2) Simply breathe and relax for a few moments to get into a meditative mind-set. Many people do this with the mindfulness breathing technique mentioned above.

3) Once in a meditative state, begin slowly, mentally counting each inhalation/exhalation series, until you reach 21 repetitions.

4) Repeat the slow cycle of mental counting of 21 breathing repetitions a total of five times.

5) When this is done, the koan is introduced and repeated over and over for as long as the meditation lasts.

For more information: http://www.anvention.com/?q=zazen

CHAKRA MEDITATION—Many of the forms of meditation were developed from the ancient yogic practices of India. Chakra mediation is a more recent practice developed by the late Paramahansa Yogananda. (If you have not read his book Autobiography of a Yogi, I highly recommend it.)

Yogananda is credited with bringing yoga and meditation to the West in 1920 and forever changing how Americans view themselves and others. His chakra meditation focuses on all the chakras (energy centers) in the body, from the base of the spine to the tip of the head. This meditative technique is

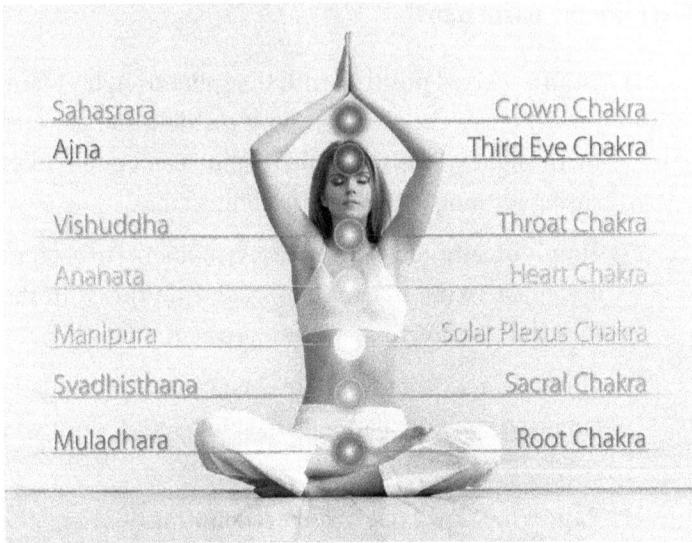

Sahasrara	Crown Chakra
Ajna	Third Eye Chakra
Vishuddha	Throat Chakra
Anahata	Heart Chakra
Manipura	Solar Plexus Chakra
Svadhisthana	Sacral Chakra
Muladhara	Root Chakra

couched in yogic language and concepts. These days, there are many variations.

Here are the basic steps:

1) Close your eyes and bring your attention inward to the inner love and peace of your heart.

2) Visualize each chakra, one at a time, and breathe with it several times as you make your way from the lower root chakra to the upper crown chakra and back down through all seven chakras.

3) Visualize and feel that the crown chakra is filled with the light and love of the Creator. Visualize this light and love as reaching out and connecting with the crown chakras of millions of others worldwide.

4) Repeat the above for each chakra in the series of seven from crown to root. Often specific prayers are recited mentally during this process.

5) On completion of the entire series, finish by chanting "Om" three times.

For more information: http://www.yogananda-srf.org

JAPA MEDITATION—The meditation method known as Japa was developed in India about 2300 B.C. As the self-help guru Wayne Dyer describes, this meditation helps you "get into the gap" by activating the sound "Ahhh." The "Ahhh" sound is found in the phonetic pronunciation of the names of the creators or gods, whether your belief in a creator is Eastern or Western. Think of the sounds made when saying the names God, Buddha, Allah, Brahman, Atman, Ra, Jehovah and others. The sound "Ahhh," like "Om," is universally believed to hold great meditative power.

Here are the basic steps:

1) Close your eyes and visualize the letters of the alphabet, one at a time, from letters A to G.

2) As you visualize each letter, say the word "Ahhh" or say the god name you prefer that stems from your belief system.

3) After visualizing the letter A and making the sound "Ahhh" on long exhale, visualize the letter B next to it. Inhale and visualize the letter B.

4) 4While visualizing the letter B, exhale while making the "Ahhh" sound.

5) Next, inhale and focus on the space (the gap) between the letters A and B and repeat the process.

6) Next, return to the letter B and again repeat the process.

7) Now visualize the letter C as standing in a row next to A and B. And repeat as above for all letters through G.

8) When your mind drifts, bring your attention back to the sound of Japa, the sound of "Ahhh."

For more information: http://www.project-meditation.org/ mt/japa_meditation.html

MINDFULNESS—Mindfulness meditation is a simple and powerful method to use for beginners and its general method is outlined here. It is best to find a quiet space and a block of time in which you will not be disturbed. Wear loose- fitting clothing and be sure to relieve yourself before you begin. You should also not be too hungry nor too full, but comfortably satisfied and at ease. Here's how to do it:

Here are the basic steps:

1) Sit or lie down in a comfortable position that allows your spine to be straight and your head aligned with it.

2) Close your eyes and take a few deep breaths to ease into the moment and begin to relax.

3) Focus your attention on your breath as it passes the tip of your nose.

4) As you inhale, merely OBSERVE, without mental comment, the sensation you feel as air passes the tip of your nose.

5) As you exhale, merely OBSERVE, without mental comment, the sensation you feel as air passes the tip of your nose.

6) When thoughts enter your mind, do not engage them, do not pass judgment on them. Merely ACKNOWLEDGE that they are there and return to observing the sensation of the breath on the tip of the nose.

In the beginning you may experience the following: A tendency to fall asleep; a mind that appears to race more than usual (it probably isn't, but your senses are closed so you just notice it more); legs that may fall asleep or tingle from poor flexibility or cramping; a tendency to unknowingly lose focus of your breathing and find that your mind has wandered to another part of your body or to a drifting thought. All of this is all okay... don't stress over it.

FOCUS ON THE PROCESS

Regardless of which meditation method you engage in, the process is the important thing. In the beginning, you may experience a tendency to fall asleep, or your mind may appear to race more than usual. Don't get discouraged.

There are many benefits to the daily practice of meditation including improved concentration, enhanced focus, unshakable emotions, inner fortitude, understanding of the self, objectivity, concentrated decision- making power and peace of mind. Physiologically, you will experience a decrease in blood pressure, respiration and metabolism, the nervous systems calm, hormones and chemicals balance and the body can return to its natural harmonious state of homeostasis.

Meditation is intended to bring you into the moment, to induce the relaxation response and to calm your bodily functions and thoughts — all to bring peace of mind and awareness of body. Even the simplest techniques, for even a few minutes each day, can make a difference in your life, in your health and in your well-being. Take some time and investigate the methods mentioned above and other methods, too. Reach out to local meditation groups and see which place and methods resonates with you. Then give it a try.

STUDY: Meditation Causes Cardiovascular and Neurological Changes

Research from Harvard-affiliated researchers at Massachusetts General Hospital (MGH)[14] shows that practicing meditation regularly for as little as eight weeks can cause beneficial physiological structural changes in the brain's grey matter. This is important because most of the brain's neural cell bodies are found within grey matter, which itself encompasses regions of the brain that effect sensory perception (sight and sound), muscle control, memory, emotions, auditory functions and how we make decisions and apply self-control. In other words, this is amazing proof of the power of meditation to positively affect almost every aspect of your well-being.

For the study the researchers utilized magnetic resonance imaging (MRI) to gain images of participants' brains two weeks before and then right after the meditation study period. For eight weeks participants (meditation experts and novices) meditated using the MBSR (mindfulness-based stress reduction) method for 27 minutes per day using guided meditation recordings.

All participants self-reported feeling less stressed. Importantly, the MRIs showed a clear decrease of the grey matter in the parts of the brain known as the amygdalae (which help us deal with stress, anxiety and controls the 'fight or flight' response). Additionally, the MRI showed an increase of gray matter in the hippocampus (the area that controls memory, learning, self-awareness, compassion).

This is objective proof that meditation changes our brains in a positive way that helps us reduce our stress response while increasing our concentration, decision making, and compassion toward others.

Another study, published in *Frontiers of Human Neuroscience*,[15] shows the benefits that long-term meditation practice has on the heart and nervous system. For the study, researchers used wireless sensor technology to examine variations between novice and experienced participants while meditating, through continuous monitoring of vital signs (via EEG, blood pressure, heart rate variability).

Forty participants (half with experience and half novice) took part in a one-week wellness retreat where their meditation sessions were monitored on their first and last days to compare changes in vital signs readings. Changes in EEG, BP and HRV showed that meditation does, objectively, produce improved physiologic responses in the body.

QIGONG: THE BREATH OF HEALTH

Qigong is the name given to ancient Chinese systems of breath work and energy cultivation. Qigong exercises balance energy in the body through coordination of thought, breath and movement. The nucleus of qigong is the exercise of consciousness and vital energy. The goal being to circulate, build and balance qi (vital energy) throughout the body to promote physical and mental health. When energy is enhanced, blockages (stagnations) of blood, oxygen and nutrients to the cells are removed and toxins can release.

With this enhanced function comes restored liver function and lower blood pressure. Regular practice of qigong exercises aid in regulating the functions of the central nervous system. Along with exercising and controlling one's mind and body, qigong influences one's physical states and pathological conditions, including high blood pressure.

When practicing qigong exercises, it is essential that you remain relaxed and focused throughout each breath. Breathe slowly and steadily while expanding and contracting the respective areas of the body, as dictated by the exercise.

Below I share two simple qigong exercises that help reduce the effects of stress and high blood pressure.

QI BALL EXERCISE—This exercise teaches you how to feel, circulate and control the flow of qi (energy) between your hands. The hands are the easiest place to begin experiencing the qi energy and, since feeling is believing, it is a good place to start.

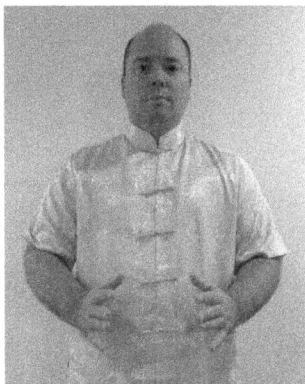

Here are the basic steps:

1) Begin by closing your eyes, relaxing your respiration and clearing your mind.

2) Once a sensation of energy is felt between your hands, very slowly and very slightly move them apart (less than two inches) while inhaling.

3) Exhale while very slowly pushing your hands together back to their starting position.

4) Repeat for at least five minutes; longer if you can.

With your elbows bent and your arms held away from your body, configure your arms and hands as if you were holding a basketball. Hold this position while breathing into your abdomen and focusing your intention on the space between your hands—but do not move them until a sensation is felt. The sensation may be heat, tingling or heaviness.

It is important to time the full breath with the full movement, so the hands must move slowly.

The exhalation must come to an end as the hands reach their starting point. Timing of breath and movement and holding of intention in the hands is vital to the exercise.

People generally report a feeling between their hands that is akin to magnets being pushed together. There is a magnetic resistance between the hands, and this is the energy coming from the hands and meeting in the middle. The closer the hands, the more concentration of energy between them and the harder it is to close them.

You will not only increase your energy, but you will shift into a state of relaxation where stress is relieved and blood pressure is reduced.

STANDING POLE EXERCISE—The standing pole exercise aims to circulate qi (energy) throughout the body, from the bottom to the top and from the back to the front. It aids in whole- body circulation of blood and energy and stretches and adjusts 19 vertebrae—from the coccyx to T1.

Breath, mind and movement are coordinated, and all movements should be slow and steady, demonstrated here by Master FaXiang Hou.

Here are the basic steps:

1) Stand comfortably with shoulders relaxed, legs a comfortable shoulders-width apart and knees very slightly bent. Keep your arms slightly away from your torso.

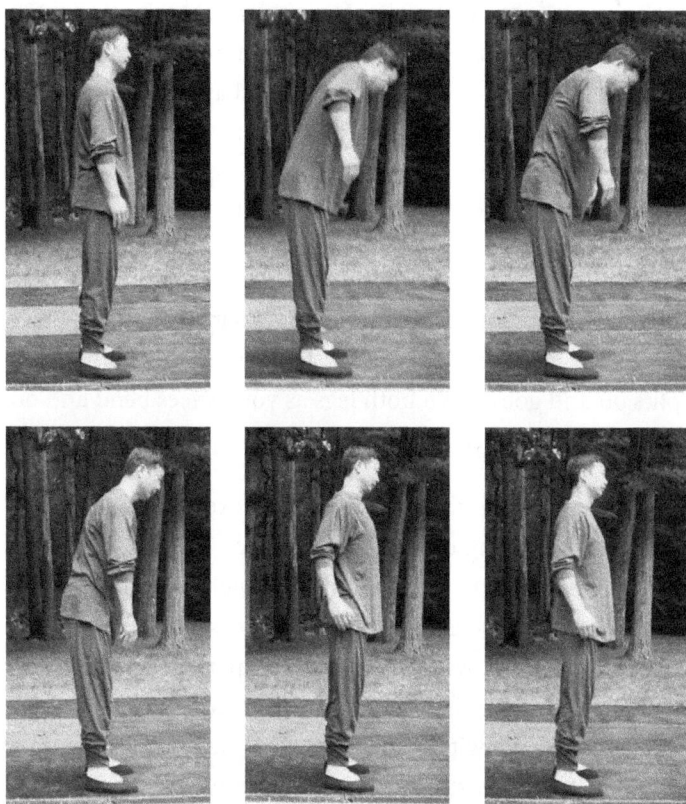

Standing Pole Exercise

2) While inhaling, concentrate on pulling qi (energy) up from the ground.

3) While exhaling, concentrate on moving the qi down your front side the moment of moving your body following the energy movement.

4) Repeat this sequence for at least five minutes, but as long as you like.

As you move up, the qi moves through your heels and up the back of your legs. As the qi passes your knees they straighten. The qi then continues past your hips up your spine to the shoulder area. When the qi reaches the base of the spine, begin to pull your shoulders up, thus moving the energy up the spine and to the top of your head. Your hips, waist and spine contract and rise as the qi moves through each area.

Follow the movement of qi from the top of your head as your shoulders move forward, down across your forehead and face, down your chest and down your stomach. At this point, the qi splits off and goes down both legs as your knees bend and out the balls of your feet.

While performing the standing pole exercise, you should experience a feeling of warmth over each area the qi travels. Be sure to keep your breath and movement coordinated and your mind on the sensation of the energy as it passes over each part of your body. With this you will experience a meditative state wherein the mind quiets down, muscles relax, and energy moves freely within the body. This state allows the body to return to homeostasis, thereby allowing the symptoms of stress to subside and blood pressure to reduce.

STUDY: Qigong Effective for Reducing the Effects of Essential Hypertension

The *American Journal of Chinese Medicine*[16] presented finds from a study designed to measure changes in blood pressure (BP), urinary catecholamines and ventilatory functions of patients with mild essential hypertension after 10 weeks of qigong.

Fifty-eight patients volunteered to participate in this study and were randomly divided into either a qigong group (n = 29), or a control group (n = 29). Systolic blood pressure and diastolic blood pressure decreased significantly in the qigong group such that both became significantly lower after 10 weeks in the qigong than in the control group.

Also, there was a significant reduction of norepinephrine, metanephrine and epinephrine compared to baseline values in the qigong group. The ventilatory functions, forced vital capacity and forced expiratory volume per sec, were increased in the qigong group, but not the control group.

These results suggest that qigong may stabilize the sympathetic nervous system, is effective in modulating levels of urinary catecholamines and BP positively and in improving ventilatory functions in mildly hyper- tensive middle-aged patients.

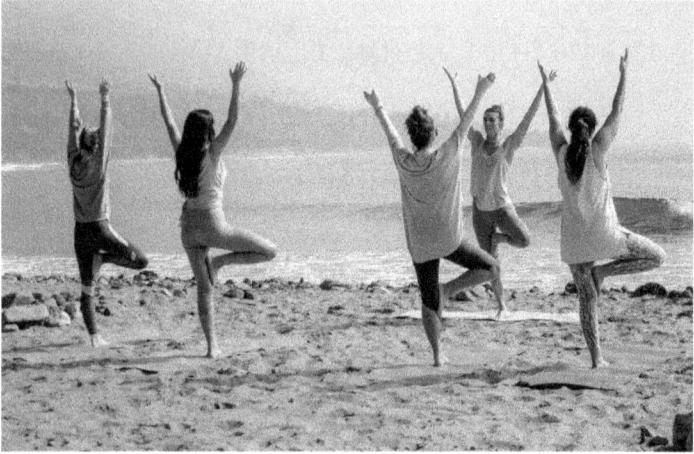

YOGA: THE POSTURE OF HEALTH

Yoga is an ancient Indian practice of health and well- being. As an exercise, it involves holding and moving between various postures, specified breathing methods and meditation. While the aim of traditional yoga is unifying mind and body with spirit, in the West it has come to be a relaxing or muscle-toning physical activity, depending on yoga style.

Regardless of which method of yoga is practiced, studies have confirmed its healing properties. In fact, many studies have found that regular practice of yoga can reduce blood pressure by as much as 15 mm/Hg. With extended practice of yoga, a level of fitness is achieved, and weight loss experienced which is also responsible for additional lowering of blood pressure.

Yoga can be an effective preventive measure and reversal mechanism of hypertension by virtue of its ability to induce a deep calming effect and slower breathing. This mechanism brings down the stress-induced fight or flight response, thereby reducing the levels of the hormones adrenaline and cortisol that are pumping through your system.

According to Dr. Sujit Chandratreya, Research Team member with Yoga Vidya Gurukul, "Regular Yoga may reduce stress hormone 'aldosterone' which is a potent vasoconstrictor (which contracts blood vessels thus increasing Blood Pressure). Preliminary studies also point out to the fact that regular yoga practice may reduce 'Vasopressin' another stress hormone secreted by pituitary gland in the brain. Vasopressin increases blood pressure. by vascular contraction."[13]

STUDY: Yoga Lowers Blood Pressure, Boost Positive Physiological Changes

Medical News Today[17] reported on several studies spanning a decade which point to its ability to reduce stress, lower blood pressure, reduce inflammation, and improve a person's quality of life.

In one study, participants had slightly or mildly elevated blood pressure and were not receiving treatment. Researchers divided them into two groups. One performed Iyengar yoga exercises for 12 weeks. The other group made personalized dietary adjustments. After comparing results, the authors concluded that "Twelve weeks of Iyengar yoga produces clinically meaningful improvements in 24-hour systolic blood pressure and diastolic blood pressure."

Another study reported on was a randomized controlled trial investigating yoga's effects on high blood pressure. It compared the effects of practicing Hatha yoga for 12 weeks with more standard approaches, and participants were randomly divided the into three groups.

The Yoga group, containing 43 people, who attended two 90-minute yoga classes each week for 12 weeks. Gradually, they also began to practice yoga at home, guided by DVD instruction.

The Healthful living group contained 48 people, who followed a health education and walking program. It included classes in nutrition and motivational guidance, and participants gradually worked up to 180 minutes of walking per week.

The Yoga-and-healthful living group contained 46 people, who attended the yoga classes and the health education and walking program, but they could opt out of home yoga.

The researchers concluded that all three approaches reduced resting blood pressure. However, at 12 weeks, the reduction in blood pressure was more significant in the group that did only yoga, compared to the group that followed the education and walking program.

There are innumerable ways in which one can benefit from the practice of mind-body exercises, like those taught in The Sedona Method™, neuro-linguistic programming, meditation, qigong and yoga. The meditative states and breathing exercises improve blood circulation and enrich the body with more red blood cells. This increases the supply of oxygen to the tissues and promotes healthier tissues and organs. The greater supply of oxygen enables the heart to pump slower while still providing enough oxygen to the body. Imbalances such as high blood pressure and rapid heart rate are made normal with prolonged, proper practice of breathing exercises.

Perhaps the most powerful effect of disciplined and prolonged practice of mind-body medicine is the ability to live in the moment. That is, removing the past and future, knowing that there is only now and that every taste, smell, task, event and thing you say or do now is all there is.

It allows you to experience life's fullest potential.

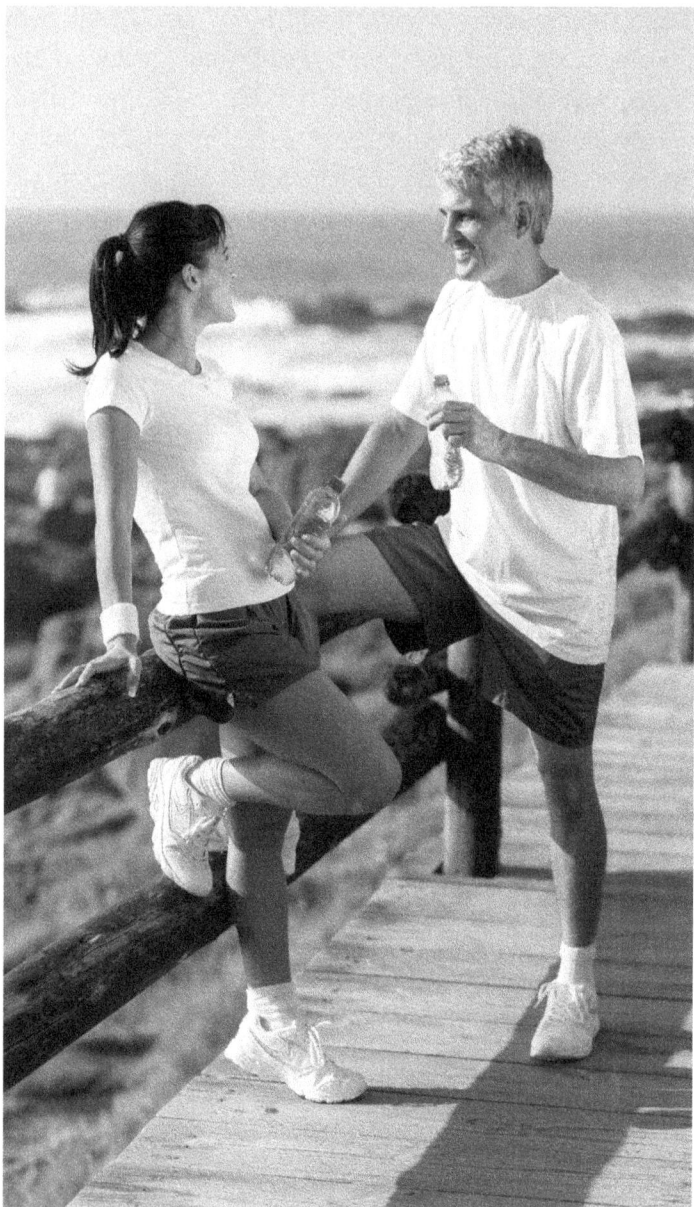

CHAPTER 4

Exercise and Blood Pressure

Exercise and blood pressure are closely related. It's no secret that regular physical activity makes the heart stronger. And a stronger heart is more able to pump blood through the body, even a sluggish one. When the heart is stronger it can do the same amount of work as a weaker heart, but with much less effort. With less effort comes a decrease on the pressure forced against the walls of your arteries… resulting in lower blood pressure.

According to the Mayo Clinic, "Becoming more active can lower your systolic blood pressure (the top number in a blood pressure reading) by an average of 5 to 10 mm/Hg. That's as good as some blood pressure medications. For some people, getting some exercise is enough to reduce the need for blood pressure medication." [18]

INCREASE YOUR PHYSICAL ACTIVITY

An on-going exercise routine also helps with body mass reduction (weight loss), which itself is a reversal and preventive measure against hypertension. Moreover, if your blood pressure is within normal ranges, exercise can help maintain it even as you age. Nothing happens overnight though, and it takes a few months of regular exercise to see a reduction in blood pressure readings.

What's more, the benefits will only remain if the exercise routine is maintained. Becoming sedentary later, all else being equal, will result again in a rise in blood pressure.

It is important to know that difficult or intense physical activity is not necessary to achieve weight loss and lower blood pressure. Engaging in regular physical activities as simple as yard work, cleaning the house, tennis, swimming, walking and Pilates do the job well.

On the contrary, too vigorous an exercise program can have adverse effects and has been shown to lead to heart disease.

VIGOROUS EXERCISE AND HEART DISEASE

In recent research coming out of New York University Medical Center,[19] it is suggested that the more often one engages in vigorous exercise the greater their risk of developing atrial fibrillation (AF). AF is a condition characterized by irregular, rapid heart rate and affects people in many ways, from simple fainting to heart failure and stroke!

In the study, participants were divided into two groups: An exercise group and a non-exercise group. Men who exercised long or hard enough to break a sweat five to seven days per week increased their chances of developing AF by an enormous 20%! And the non- exercise control group? No increase in their propensity for AF was reported.

The big surprise is this: The participants who were in the "break a sweat" group were deemed to be "healthy." It was made up of men under the age of 50 who run on a regular basis. Common sense would say the opposite results should be the case. But the study clearly shows that the incidence of atrial fibrillation in men who jog increased by a massive 50%! And it was up by 74% in young men who break a sweat on a regular basis! For those who run marathons, training for them from between 10 and 19 hours per week, the *British Medical Journal* (BMJ) reported study results supporting the negative association of vigorous exercise and heart disease.[20] The *American Journal of Cardiology* also reported study results on the adverse effects of strenuous exercise and heart disease.[21]

By now, you may be worried about your own condition. However, it seems that AF is common and even expected in so-called healthy athletes. This is the case because cardiomegaly (enlargement of the heart) is so common in athletes that doctors don't even tell them they have a condition that can lead to heart disease. Yet in normal, non-athletic people, if their electrocardiograms showed these same signs, the doctors would be very concerned and would let them know!

The long and short is this: The essence of the study indicates that breaking a sweat on a regular basis is bad for your heart. And history shows that marathoners and other top athletes die at a young age as a result of heart disease. And in China, where tai chi and qigong are practiced by millions, heart disease and young heart-related deaths are amongst the world's lowest rates. Below, we'll look at one exercise that offers big rewards but asks for little exertion in return.

THE STANDING HEALTH EXERCISE

In my search for the best in holistic medicine I have traveled the globe and spent time with healers of all types: Shamans, psychic surgeons, qigong masters, faith healers, herbalists, bone setters… you name it. While studying a method of qigong in Asia known as Zhan Zhuang ("Pile Standing"), my teacher told me something very strange.

"This neigong (internal) exercise forces you to stand still and not move for a long time. Because of this, your energy will increase, your body will warm, and your muscles will strengthen. But you will not damage your joints from excessive movement, nor tax your heart through robust movement, nor damage the lungs through too rapid respiration."[22]

I have to say that I had trouble swallowing this last part and for the past 25 years I have been trying to reason it out in my mind… why not increase heart rate and respiration? After all, isn't the entire fitness industry in the Western world based on elevating heart rate, increasing lung capacity and burning calories from sweating and muscle strength development?

Well, like with so many other things, it looks like the ancient Chinese knew what they were talking about. As the *BMJ* and *AMS* studies indicated, there is a risk of heart disease from vigorous exercise.

Since "pile standing" is a simple exercise that requires only the space of standing, it is perfect for the busy person suffering from hypertension who also has no time to memorize new exercise routines or go to a Pilates class.

This practice is as easy as:

1) Standing with your legs a shoulder's width apart

2) Bending the knees only one-to-two-inches

3) Bending both arms and holding them at the same level. Following are two standing postures for you to do in sequence or on alternating days if you want to mix things up.

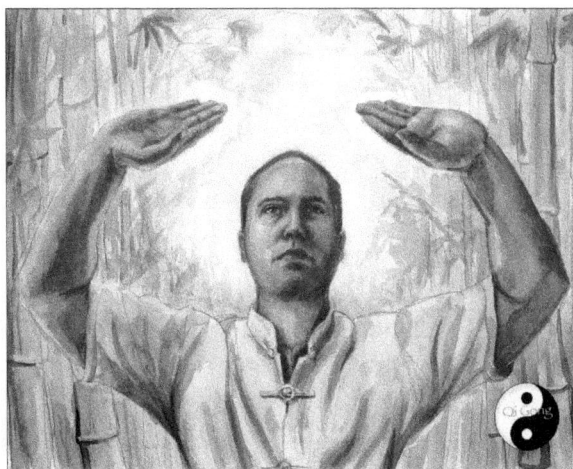

For the first posture, stand as described above, with both arms held out at the sides, elbows bent slightly, forearms parallel to the ground and palms facing down. Try to imagine that your palms are floating on water. And don't move a muscle!

Once the posture is assumed, quiet the mind by not stressing over distracting thoughts that may come—simply allow them to go freely without judgment.

Next, regulate respiration by quietly breathing in and out at a steady relaxed pace. Now enjoy yourself for the next 10 to 20 minutes.

You'll be surprised to find how difficult merely standing still can be, but you'll derive numerous benefits as a result.

For the second posture, stand as described above while holding the arms in front of you, elbows bent at chest level, palms facing your body. It's like you're hugging a tree.

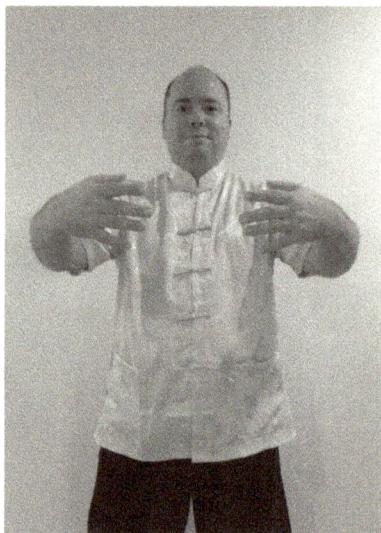

Don't move a muscle!

Once the posture is assumed, quiet the mind by not stressing over distracting thoughts that may come— simply allow them to go freely without judgment.

Next, regulate respiration by quietly breathing in and out at a steady relaxed pace.

Now enjoy yourself for the next 10 to 20 minutes.

Again, you'll be surprised to find how difficult merely standing still can be.

You see, while it appears as if you are doing nothing at all, the body is engaged in a process of physical activity. While quieting the mind and regulating respiration you are reducing stress, relaxing the cerebral cortex and rejuvenating the central nervous system. You are also working muscles by virtue of maintaining an isometric posture wherein the knees and elbows are bent, and the arms are raised. This must be held steady without release until the end of the session. This elevates heart rate without overtaxing the heart, improves the circulation of blood and oxygen throughout the body and increases metabolic functions while releasing toxins and tension from the body.

WALK YOUR WAY TO LOWER BLOOD PRESSURE

If done correctly, brisk walking can be one of the safest, most beneficial and enjoyable exercises for anyone. Walking is an aerobic activity, but since it is low-impact there is little wear-and-tear on the joints and little (if any) triggering of pain from the jarring action of the body often experienced in high-impact aerobic exercise or jogging.

Although it is a simple activity, walking actually utilizes most of the muscles of the body to propel you forward and keep you on balance while increasing respiration, heart and lung function, blood and oxygen flow and the "burning off" of blood sugars and fats and removal of toxins and other wastes through sweat and improved eliminative functions.

Walking is indeed simple and ordinary. Yet in one 30-minute session you can raise HDL (good cholesterol) levels, increase respiration within safe limits, sweat out toxins, release endorphins (the feel-good hormone), improve heart function, begin reducing weight, reduce stress, promote relaxation and improve overall endurance and body tone. All of these have a positive overall effect on blood pressure.

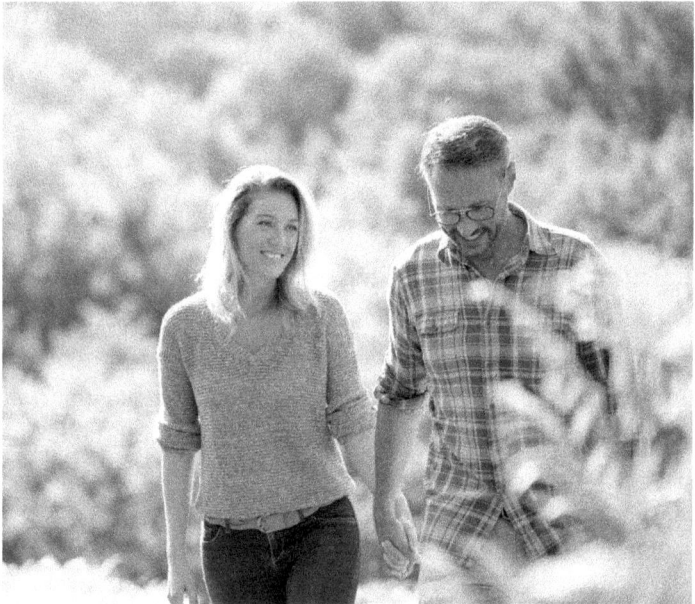

Whether it's walking, standing, Pilates or yard work, exercise is an essential part of any hypertension reversal and prevention program. Here's what Arthur Agatston, MD, author of *The South Beach Diet*,[23] says about it:

> *"Exercise lowers your blood pressure and increases your good cholesterol. Exercise regularly and eat properly and you're doing just about all you can to ensure a healthy cardiac future. You're already doing far more for yourself than medical science can do for you."*

So, go ahead and take a brisk 30-minute walk and later that day or the next day, stand still for 30 minutes. You may never feel as good as this.

STUDY: A Little Walking Cuts Blood Pressure

A study reported in WebMD Health News[24] shows that even a little bit of weekly exercise is enough to lower blood pressure and improve overall fitness.

In the study, published in the Journal of Epidemiology and Community Health, researchers invited 106 healthy but sedentary civil servants to take part in an exercise program for 12 weeks. About a third were told to briskly walk for 30 minutes, five days a week. Another third was told to briskly walk for 30 minutes a day, three days a week; the remaining third were told not to change their sedentary lifestyle at all.

The participants wore pedometers to monitor their walking and researchers measured their blood pressure, blood cholesterol, weight, hip and waist size and overall fitness before and after the study.

The results showed systolic (the top number) blood pressure dropped—and waist and hip measurements shrunk significantly—in both the three-day-a-week and five-day-a-week exercise groups.

Systolic blood pressure dropped by five points among those who exercised three days a week and by six points among those who exercised five days a week.

Waist and hip measurements fell by 2.6 centimeters and 2.4 centimeters respectively among the three-day-a-week exercisers and by 2.5 centimeters and 2.2 centimeters among the five-day-a-week exercise group.

CHAPTER 5

Diet and Hypertension

Dietary changes must be a central component of any hypertension reduction and prevention strategy. For many patients, particularly those who are diabetic or pre-diabetic, diet needs to be the fundamental focus, as correcting poor food choices is the easiest piece of the program to get a handle on. It may be difficult to remember to breathe and meditate when stressed but choosing whole grain over white bread is a visual choice that is before your eyes.

For the purposes of lowering high blood pressure and not making it worse through your eating choices, the information presented in this section is broad based. That is, there is not a specific diet with necessary measurements or caloric requirements to remember. Instead, we look at foods that clinical trials have shown to cause hypertension (such as salt, fructose, high fructose corn syrup and sugar) and those shown to decrease hypertension (such as vitamin D, chili peppers, beets and watermelon). We then provide an overview of the hypertension diet that is the most widely accepted and adopted by the leading health associations in the country.

Where food is concerned it is clear-cut which ones need to be avoided and which should be center stage in your diet. By following these guidelines, your blood pressure will drop back to within normal ranges and eating will no longer be a cause of concern for your overall health.

REDUCE YOUR SALT CONSUMPTION

Salt is the arch enemy of normal blood pressure. When we consume too much sodium, our body retains too much water. This increase in water retention increases our overall circulatory volume, which is the load our blood vessels must handle when doing their job. Just like lifting a heavier object increases the load on our arms and strains our muscles, this fluid load increases the strain on our heart and blood vessels. Increased strain and pressure cause hypertension.

When doing some additional research for this book I investigated dozens of studies and articles, from the academic to the more popular. I was amazed at how many Internet writers dismissed the role of salt in raising blood pressure, given the abundance of clinical trials that clearly point to a direct connection between the two. While we know why salt causes blood pressure to rise, it is only from recent studies that scientists understand how salt adversely affects blood pressure.

Scientists from the United States and Japan have uncovered the physiological process that explains how salt raises blood

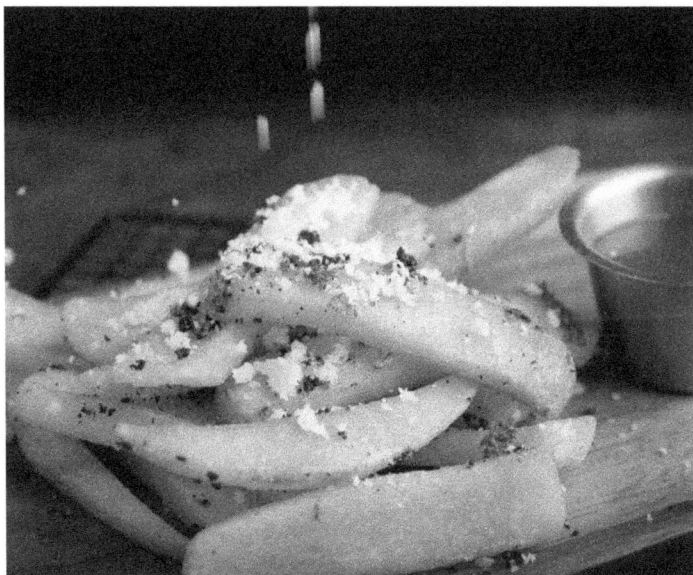

pressure. According to the study, available on the University of Maryland website, it has something to do with a hormone known as ouabain that is secreted by the adrenal gland. The information to the right is extracted from that study and explains the process in detail.

Total sodium intake must be reduced to help reverse and prevent hypertension. The easiest way to begin reducing salt intake is to stop adding it as seasoning to foods after they have been prepared. In other words, some salt for cooking as usual but then no extra salt added at the table (or restaurant) once the food is served. Once you get used to that reduction, then you can reduce the amount of salt you use while cooking or preparing foods. What's more, simply choosing "low salt" versions of your favorite snacks, like pretzels or chips, is another fast way to reduce salt consumption right away without completely changing your eating habits all at once... which is often the cause of failure of most diets.

STUDY: The Pump, the Exchanger, and the Holy Spirit

According to findings published in *Cell Physiology*,[25] eating excess salt stimulates the secretion of too much ouabain (pronounced wah-bane) — a naturally occurring hormone secreted by the adrenal gland. The hormone has a dramatic effect on two proteins that together, regulate the amount of sodium and calcium within the smooth muscle cells of the arteries.

The first protein, known as the Alpha-2 Sodium Pump, is responsible for removing excess sodium from artery cells. The second protein, called the Sodium-Calcium Exchanger, replaces sodium with calcium. The proteins, located in the cell membrane, work together to maintain a healthy balance of sodium and calcium inside the cell. Researchers in Baltimore and Ohio determined that the Alpha-2 Sodium Pump in artery muscle cells is the target of ouabain's action.

Excess ouabain upsets the balance by disabling the Sodium Pump, causing sodium to accumulate in artery cells. The additional sodium causes the Sodium Calcium

Exchanger protein to bring in too much calcium, which triggers artery constriction and hypertension. "The process that leads to high blood pressure is a vicious cycle," says Mordecai P. Blaustein, MD. "Too much sodium in the blood stimulates ouabain secretion. The ouabain interacts with the Sodium Pump, causing sodium and calcium to accumulate in the cells."

NOT ALL SUGARS ARE CREATED EQUAL

In research published in the journal *Open Heart*,[26] scientists found that fructose was the worst culprit among HBP causative factors. The reason is that fructose is the sugar most found within our processed and packaged foods and drinks. While sucrose is also found in these food sources, it is made up of equal parts fructose and glucose. However, high fructose corn syrup is often made up of 55% fructose to 45% glucose, but its ratio can skew as much as 80/20. This makes it nearly twice the fructose as sucrose (table sugar) and much more difficult for the body to metabolize.

According to the research report, "evidence from epidemiological studies and experimental trials in animals and humans suggests that added sugars, particularly fructose, may increase blood pressure and blood pressure variability, increase heart rate and myocardial oxygen demand, and contribute to inflammation, insulin resistance and broader metabolic dysfunction."[27]

When we consider obesity, metabolic syndrome and systemic inflammation as among the killers of quality of life, do we need more evidence to cut out packaged foods and drinks and go natural?

While it is hoped that the research on added fructose to packaged foods and drinks will steer you clear of them, don't let the information keep you from eating sugars in their natural state. While the researchers found a direct correlation between consumption of "added" fructose to packaged foods and a rise in high blood pressure, no such correlation was found between naturally accruing sugar (including fructose) in whole fresh foods.

It seems that when the natural sugars found in fruits and vegetables is in its natural state—with accompanying water, fiber, fats, carbohydrates, and other elements—the body can digest and process it effectively. This fact was most evident when a trial was conducted wherein participants switched from a typical Western diet to one containing an impressive 20 servings of whole fruit, actually saw a significant decrease "in systolic blood pressure, despite a fructose intake of approximately 200g."

LIMIT YOUR INTAKE OF FRUCTOSE

Fructose is a simple sugar, or monosaccharide, that is derived from fruits and vegetables. In doses that are naturally consumed while eating unprocessed whole fruits and vegetables, fructose is safe for your body. However, in high doses like those found in processed foods and beverages, fructose has been linked to increased blood pressure. In fact, a new study finds that a diet high in fructose increases the risk of hypertension or high blood pressure.

Over the last century, processed food purveyors have begun adding more simple sugars to their products to add flavor. During this period the number of Americans suffering from high blood pressure has skyrocketed.

A study presented at the American Society of Nephrology's 42nd Annual Meeting found that the rate of obesity has increased sharply since the development of high fructose corn syrup (HFCS) and that the prevalence of HFCS in processed foods may have something to do with it. It's been reported that Americans now consume 30% more fructose than they did 20 years ago.

The study showed that a diet of more than 74 grams of fructose a day led to dramatic increases in risk of hypertension for those with slightly higher blood pressure. Participants who had a blood pressure level of 160/100 had an 87% higher risk of developing hypertension. The adverse is also true. Wherein consuming more fructose can raise blood pressure, reducing its consumption has also been clinically proven to lower blood pressure.

STUDY: Lower Blood Pressure by Cutting Fructose

Results of a University of Colorado at Denver study[27] suggest that hypertensive individuals may be able to naturally lower their blood pressure by consuming a diet low in added fructose. For the study, lead author Diana Jalal, MD, and her colleagues from the university's Health Sciences Center, recruited nearly 4,600 adults over the age of 18 and had them fill out dietary questionnaires regarding their average daily consumption of processed fruit juices, soft drinks, bakery products and candy.

After taking into account other risk factors the researchers found that individuals who consumed more than 72 grams of fructose each day were between 26% and 77% (depending upon the blood pressure threshold) more likely to be hypertensive than those who eat few foods containing added sugar.

As part of your program for reducing and preventing high blood pressure it is important to avoid consuming foods high in fructose and high fructose corn syrup. While it is best to read the labels of foods before buying or consuming them, here is a list of foods that are generally found to be high in fructose: Breakfast Cereals, Processed Baked Goods, Fruit Snacks and Juices, Canned Soups, Packaged Sauces and Gravies, Processed cookies and sweets, diet beverages.

CONSUME FEWER SOFT DRINKS

Individuals who are looking to lower their blood pressure without taking medication may be able to do so by moderately reducing their intake of sugar-sweetened beverages, according to a new study.

For the 18-month study, which was published in the Journal of the American Heart Association, a research team from the Louisiana State University Health Science Center recruited 810 adults with early stage hypertension who drank an average of 11 ounces of sugary beverages each day, well below the American average of 23 daily ounces.[28]

At the end of the study, participants who reduced their soft drink intake by at least half lowered their systolic blood

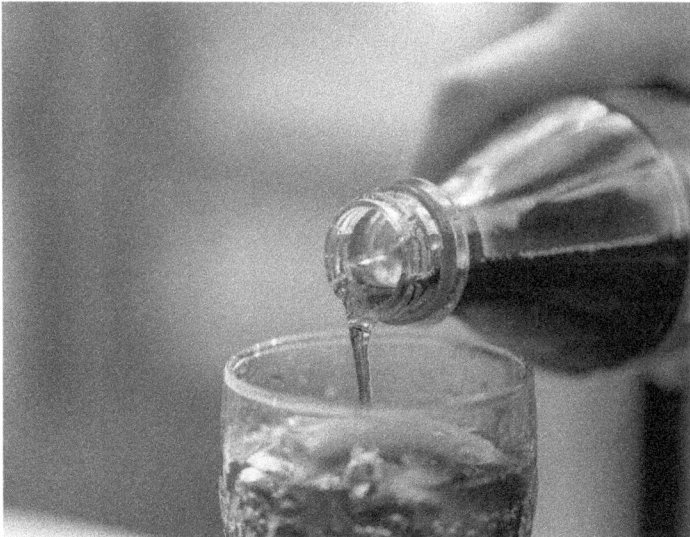

pressure by an average of 1.8 points and their diastolic blood pressure by 1.1 points.

"We found a direct dose-response relationship," said study leader Liwei Chen. "Individually, it was not a big reduction. But population-wise, reducing total consumption could have a huge impact."

According to background information included in the report, a three-point reduction in blood pressure can lower heart disease mortality risk by as much as 5%.

The correlation between lower blood pressure and reduced soft drink intake remained after accounting for weight loss and other risk factors. If ever there were more reason to stop drinking soft drinks than weight loss and chemical toxins, the ability to lower blood pressure by avoiding them is it!

BEET HIGH BLOOD PRESSURE

Research from Barts and The London School of Medicine and Dentistry[29] has shown that consuming beetroot juice can drop your blood pressure by 10 mmHg. This decreased pressure effect was shown to last a whopping 24 hours. That means that one cup of beetroot juice daily may help keep your blood pressure within normal range or closer to it.

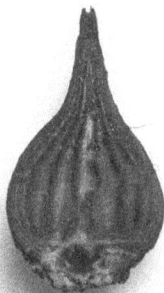

The Beetroot Study

During this research, scientists gathered 15 participants who all had systolic blood pressure (the top number) between 140-159 mmHg. They had no other health concerns and were not on medication for blood pressure. They were asked to drink 250ml (8oz) of beetroot juice or water containing a low amount of nitrate for 24 hours. During that time, their blood pressure was measured and observed.

Their blood pressure dropped an average of 10 mmHg within a few hours. Positive results were still evident the next day.

The scientists believe that nitrate in the beetroot juice caused the beneficial drop. About 0.2 grams of dietary nitrate is contained in one cup of beetroot juice. (It's also found in a large bowl of lettuce.) Nitrate causes a widening of blood vessels that allows blood to flow more easily, thus reducing pressure. Nitrates are used in drugs used to treat angina, and they are absorbed from soil into vegetables through their roots. Vegetables known to be high in nitrate include beetroot, fennel, cabbage and lettuce.

Researcher Amrita Ahluwalia said: "We were surprised by how little nitrate was needed to see such a large effect. This study shows that compared to individuals with healthy blood pressure much less nitrate is needed to produce the kinds of decreases in blood pressure that

> might provide clinical benefits in people who need to lower their blood pressure. However, we are still uncertain as to whether this effect is maintained in the long term."

While it is not yet known whether nitrate consumption through vegetables like beetroot can lead to long-term corrections in blood pressure without lifestyle changes, it does point to a fast and natural way to lower blood pressure daily. This is a boon for those suffering this nasty condition and the symptoms associated with it.

My simple advice for HBP sufferers: Drink a cup of beetroot juice daily, reduce salt consumption by 1,000 mg per day and practice daily meditation or relaxation practices. These three things, simple, inexpensive and holistic, are not that difficult to achieve. If you can manage a few daily changes, you may be able to control this life-threatening disease and avoid being one of its statistics.

ENJOY SOME WATERMELON

A new study published in the *American Journal of Hypertension* suggests that watermelon may be a factor in combating hypertension.[30] Arturo Figueroa, the study's lead investigator, said that the research team discovered that watermelon, "may prevent prehypertension from progression to full-blown hypertension, a major risk factor for heart attacks and strokes."

For the study, the scientists used an amino acid, L-citrulline, which they extracted from watermelons. This extract was administered every day for six weeks to nine patients with high blood pressure.

As a result, all the participants were able to lower their blood pressure. Arterial function was also improved in these individuals. Meanwhile, none of the subjects reported experiencing any side effects after taking the extract.

The researchers noted that watermelon also provides other nutrients, including vitamins A, B6, C and a powerful antioxidant known as lycopene. In turn, this may lead to improving the symptoms of other diseases. Figueroa added that individuals who have been diagnosed with Type 2 diabetes could also benefit from either watermelon extracts or this food in its natural form.

GOTTA LOVE THE GARLIC

Garlic has been hailed for centuries as an effective medicinal herb. Its benefits include boosting immunity, curing E. coli, reducing infections, scaring away vampires and lowering blood pressure. Kidding aside, garlic has been shown clinically to promote and support heart and blood health in those suffering from heart-related problems including high blood pressure, high cholesterol, coronary heart disease, heart attack and atherosclerosis (hardening of the arteries).

In fact, research indicates that in people with hypertension, garlic can reduce their blood pressure by as much as 8%.

Research published in the journal *Integrated Blood Pressure Control*,[31] points to garlic supplements showing promise in the treatment of uncontrolled hypertension, lowering blood pressure (BP) by about 10 mmHg systolic and 8 mmHg diastolic.

According to the researchers, the standardizable and highly tolerable aged garlic extract has the potential to lower BP in hypertensive individuals similarly to standard BP medication, via biologically plausible mechanisms of action.

Primarily, polysulfides in garlic have the potential to upregulate H_2S production via enzymatic and nonenzymatic pathways, which promote vasodilation and BP reduction. The polysulfides in garlic may also influence regulation of nitric oxide (NO) redox signaling pathways, including NO-mediated vasodilation and reduction of BP.

PASS THE PARMESAN, PLEASE

A specific cheese known as Grana Padano was selected for the study. Created by the Cistercian monks of Chiaravalle,

Italy, in the 12th century, Grana Padano is like Parmigiano Reggiano (popularly known as "parmesan" cheese). The grainy, granular-textured cheese is made from unpasteurized, semi-skimmed cow's milk that is aged for anywhere between nine months and up to two years.

Medpagetoday reported on the study, which was presented by Giuseppe Crippa, MD, of Guglielmo da Saliceto Hospital and Catholic University in Piacenza, Italy, at the American Society of Hypertension meeting.[32] According to a study, sprinkling a few tablespoons of this cheese on food daily lowers blood pressure an equal amount as compared to antihypertensive medications.

The trial included 30 patients with mild-to-moderate high blood pressure who, for the prior three months, had been on a daily regimen of prescription BP lowering medication. For the study, participants were randomly assigned into a double-blind, crossover design to 30g Grana Padano cheese or placebo for 2 months, with individualized dietary counseling for both groups to keep other dietary habits unchanged for the duration of the study.

According to researchers, not only did the daily cheese sprinkle work as well as the antihypertensive medications, but also beat out placebo. "A daily 30g dose of the Italian hard cheese lowered blood pressure by a mean 6/5 mm Hg more than did a placebo of shredded bread scented to mimic the cheese and with the same fat, calcium, and sodium profile."

Will this work with other cheeses? The research is unclear. It is postulated that the longer aging process of Grana Padano allows for compounds to develop that do not have time with younger cheeses. More research needs to be done. But for now, it is good news that adding sprinkles of aged Italian cheese to spaghetti or broccoli or salads daily will help lower blood pressure.

ENJOY SOME CINNAMON

Loaded with antioxidants, cinnamon is great for cardiovascular health. Studies show consumption of cinnamon is associated with a notable reduction in blood pressure, especially in those who are also prediabetic or have type II diabetes. Cinnamon also helps reduce cholesterol and clear arterial plaque.

According to results published in the October 2013 issue of the journal *Nutrition*, short-term consumption of cinnamon is associated with "a notable reduction" in both systolic and diastolic blood pressure, especially in those who are also prediabetic or have type 2 diabetes.[33] These results came from taking 500 mg to 2.4 g of cinnamon consumed daily for 12 weeks. The researchers concluded that cinnamon made possible significant drops in blood pressure.

GET MORE POTASSIUM

The updated Dietary Guidelines for Americans that was released in 2005 shined a spotlight on potassium and its role in reducing blood pressure. The benefit of potassium on blood pressure was confirmed by the Third National Health and Nutritional Examination Survey (NHANES III).[34]

Published in the *Archives of Internal Medicine*, data on more than 17,000 adults indicated that adequate potassium intake from fruits and vegetables can lower blood pressure.

Results showed that a diet with eight and a half daily servings of fruits and vegetables (providing 4,100mg of potassium) lowered blood pressure by 7.2/2.8 mm/Hg (systolic/diastolic) in people diagnosed with high blood pressure, compared to a diet providing only three and a half servings of fruits and vegetables (providing 1,700 mg of potassium).

Potassium is readily available in healthful foods, including the following:

Apricots, Bananas, Beans, Bran Wheat, Currents, Figs, Gammon, Muesli, Nuts, Tofu, Tomato Puree, Raisins, Potatoes, Seeds, Soybeans, Soya Flour, Veal, Wheat Germ.

INCREASE THE MAGNESIUM

Magnesium is essential to the proper functioning of hundreds of biochemical reactions in the body. These functions include promoting bone health, nerve and muscle function, the maintenance of steady heart rhythm, regulation of blood sugar, immune system support and the maintenance of normal blood pressure levels. Approximately 60% of the magnesium in our body is found in our bones, while 39% is in our cells and a mere 1% in our blood.

While hundreds of clinical studies espouse the need for magnesium, almost 70% of Americans do not get enough in their daily diet. The recommended daily allowance (RDA) is between 300 mg/day and 400 mg/day. However, dieticians recommend nearly twice that number. Either way, it seems American women are only consuming 200 mg/day and American men only 250 mg/day.

But consumption of too little magnesium is only half the issue. Our common diet, which is high in fat, suppresses the body's natural ability to absorb magnesium. And insufficient magnesium consumption, or adequate consumption with poor absorption, can raise cholesterol, which leads to high blood pressure. However, since magnesium is utilized in the production of the vasodilator prostaglandin E1, it helps blood vessels relax and widen, allowing a freer flow of blood and lowering blood pressure.

By reducing your overall fat consumption and increasing your consumption of magnesium rich food sources, you can begin lowering high blood pressure and working toward its prevention. Magnesium is readily available in healthful foods including the following:

Black Beans, Lima Beans, Soy Milk, Raw Broccoli, Nuts, Peas, Seeds, Spinach, Squash, Halibut, Whole Grains, Rockfish, Scallops, Okra, Oysters.

ADOPT THE DASH DIET PLAN

Diet fads come and go with each passing year. Some are based on solid research and some are based on gimmicks. The problems with most diets are that they are either unrealistic in their caloric restriction or, because they are only concerned with weight loss, they are not altogether healthy. But there is one dietary program that is different because it is easy to follow, healthy, provides lots of tasty options and it is proven to reverse hypertension.

An acronym for Dietary Approaches to Stop Hypertension, the DASH diet plan has been proven to reduce blood pressure in studies carried out by the National Institutes of Health (NIH). Moreover, it was developed by the National Heart, Lung and Blood Institute (part of the United States Department of Health and Human Services) and is endorsed by the American Heart Association.

In targeting hypertension, DASH is constructed around low salt consumption. More than that, it is extremely nutritionally dense and healthful. It endorses the consumption of fresh fruit, vegetables, low-fat dairy, whole grain products, nuts, fish, poultry and foods rich in potassium, magnesium and calcium. At the same time, it espouses reducing the intake of foods that are high in fat, saturated fat and cholesterol, sweets and red meat.

Like any diet, for DASH to be optimally effective one must consume daily serving amounts from each of the food groups allowed while reducing salt, fat and sugar consumption over time. Basic tenets of DASH suggest beginning by adding

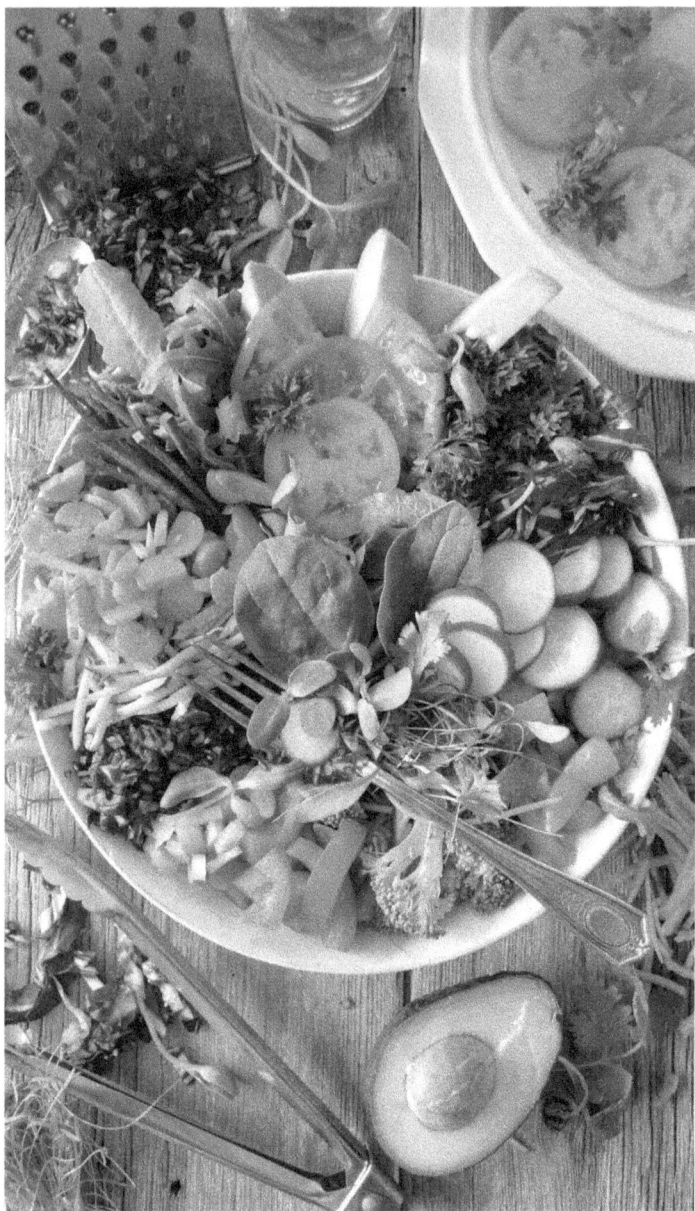

servings of vegetables to your lunch and dinner and eating fruit between meals while at the same time reducing the use of butter, margarine and salad dressings while consuming low-fat dairy three times per day. Meat is limited to six ounces per day, while snacks are confined to unsalted pretzels, nuts, graham crackers, fat-free yogurt, popcorn and raw vegetables.

There are so many terrific things about this diet, the least of which, for our purposes here, is that it proves in clinical studies to reduce high blood pressure in as little as two weeks. I suggest you take a few moments and get better acquainted with DASH by visiting their website at www.DashDiet.org

EAT FROM THE SOURCE

Cardiovascular disease is preventable and, in many cases, reversible — and diet plays an important role. Having a healthy long life may just be a matter of consuming more heart-healthy foods. You can lower blood pressure, reduce bad cholesterol and reduce the burden on the cardiovascular system with the right food. One of the best prescriptions I know of is to make sure, of the food you eat, that most of it comes from this list:

Asparagus — Because asparagus is high in fiber, minerals and vitamins B1, B2, C, E, K, it can naturally reduce inflammation, lower blood pressure, and prevent blood clots. For those who love asparagus, enjoy! For others like me, who can't stand the smell or taste, there are plenty other foods to replace it with!

Avocados — While technically a fruit, many consider avocado a vegetable. But it doesn't matter because this savory delight can lower bad (LDL) cholesterol while improving good (HDL) cholesterol to improve heart health. Consuming just one avocado daily for a week can reduce your cholesterol by 17%. I eat mine right out of the skin, on sandwiches, on salads or blended in smoothies.

B Vitamins — Studies have shown the importance of B vitamins on heart health. B6, folic acid, niacin and others have been shown to reduce arterial thickness. Some of the best sources of B vitamins are poultry, seafood, bananas, leafy green vegetables such as spinach, potatoes and fortified cereals.

Broccoli — Because broccoli is high in Vitamin K it can help prevent calcium from damaging arterial walls. And because it is high in fiber, this cancer fighting vegetable also reduces blood pressure and cholesterol.

Chia seeds — High in fiber and ALA (alpha-linolenic acid), these seeds can lower blood pressure, triglycerides (fat), and cholesterol. All essential for improved heart function.

Coconut oil —Coconut oil contains lauric acid that protects against blood coagulation and reduces risk of heart disease. It is also known to help balance cholesterol and prevent arterial plaque buildup, making this my new favorite oil. I add it to smoothies and its high burning temperature makes it perfect for cooking.

Coffee — Hundreds of new coffee studies emerge and among the most exciting are the ones showing that drinking a few cups a day can prevent onset of Parkinson's disease, reduce risk of prostate cancer, and can reduce risk of cardiovascular disease by 20%.

Cranberries — Cranberry juice was my mother's favorite beverage for decades and she swore by its healing powers. Because this berry is rich in antioxidants and helps balance cholesterol to healthy LDL/HDL levels, cranberries have been shown to reduce overall risk of heart disease by a whopping 40%.

Dark Leafy Greens — Homocysteine is a killer amino acid that is linked to higher risk of heart attack and stroke by supporting plaque formation and damage to arteries. Luckily, a few servings of dark green leafy veggies like kale and spinach (which I drink in daily smoothies) can reduce risk of heart disease by 11%.

Green Tea — Consumed throughout Asia for centuries, green tea is now becoming more popular in the West. Because it is rich in catechins, green tea helps decrease the amount of cholesterol that is absorbed by the body. Green tea improves cholesterol by reducing blood fat and arterial blockage. Green and black teas also help reduce cholesterol and risk of stroke.

Garlic — This wonder spice helps boost immunity, suppress infections, reduce arterial plaque buildup, prevent blood clots, lower cholesterol and reduce blood pressure. No wonder the Mediterranean people are so relaxed and healthy!

Nuts — Nuts may also reduce your risk of heart attack and cardiovascular disease, especially walnuts, hazelnuts, almonds, pistachios, and pecans because they are rich in **polyunsaturated** fats and can help maintain blood vessel health and reduce cholesterol.

Olive Oil — Olive oil is heart healthy because it helps reduce bad LDL cholesterol. Extra-virgin olive oil has been shown to be the most desirable as it is made from the first press of the olive and contains more antioxidants. Studies show a 41% reduction in likelihood of stroke when using olive oil daily when compared to non-users.

Omega-3 Fatty Acids —These support heart health by increasing HDL (healthy cholesterol), which helps shuttle bad cholesterol from the body. Omega-3s reduce inflammation and help lower blood pressure. They can also shrink the risk of blood clots while reducing the chances of heart disease, arthritis, and cancer. Supplementation is a great way to get more in your diet, as is eating two servings weekly of sigh like albacore tuna, halibut, herring, mackerel, wild salmon, and sardines.

Pomegranates — My wife's new food craze is eating the seeds of two pomegranates each day. And you know what, her cholesterol dropped to the lowest level of her life. Pomegranates contain tons of fiber that shuttles cholesterol out of the blood and reduces plaque buildup, and antioxidants that protect the arteries from damage. Studies also show this fruit triggers the body's production of nitric oxide, which helps to keep your blood flowing and your arteries open!

Red Wine — A glass or two per day of red wine is said to cut your risk of heart attack and stroke by as much as 50%. What's more, arterial plaque buildup is reduced over 30% in those who consume the beverage daily. Aside from being high in resveratrol and antioxidants, red wine (like pomegranates) also stimulates the body's production of nitric acid.

Turmeric — Curcumin, an active component of turmeric, is known to reduce inflammation. Inflammation is perhaps the major cause of clogged arteries. Consuming curcumin supplements or adding turmeric to your cooking (think Indian food), can reduce fatty deposits in the arteries and protect your heart.

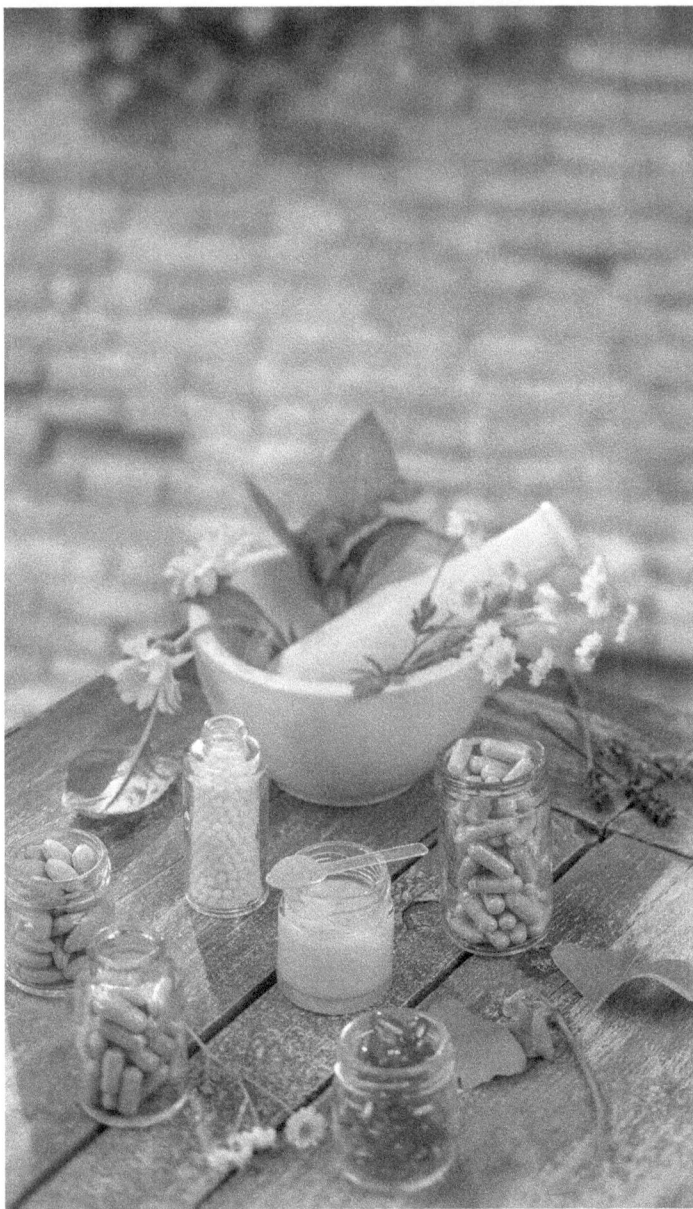

CHAPTER 6

Natural Supplements and Herbal Remedies

This section provides an idea of what natural supplements and herbal remedies are available to assist in lowering blood pressure. While these supplements are all natural and safe, they have much the same result as prescription drug therapy. That is, they temporarily reduce blood pressure and, to be effective over time, they need to be taken continually. In other words, like with prescriptions, once you stop taking these supplements their effects diminish and unless you have changed your lifestyle the hypertension will surely return.

That said, as a method to begin getting a handle on the blood pressure issue and doing so with natural ingredients while making healthy lifestyle choices, supplementation and herbal remedies provide good support.

Taking nutraceuticals, or nutritional supplements, is straight-forward. They are safe if taken in the prescribed dosages, are easily found in most drugstores and larger retail outlets and can be taken by anyone. Chinese herbal patent medicines and homeopathic remedies, on the other hand, are made to address specific sets of signs and symptoms being experienced along with hypertension. Thus, more care should be taken when selecting the right remedy with attention to detail on accompanying symptoms.

NATURAL SUPPLEMENTS

There are supplements for just about every health condition.

Yet it is always best to get your nutrients in their natural whole state in the form of food. In Chapter 6 we discussed the role of diet as part of a hypertension program. There we listed potassium, magnesium and garlic. These also come in supplement form and could have been included in this section. However, those are best consumed in their food states. Here we offer two supplements that are okay to take as supplements as well as eaten in food.

Cod Liver Oil—Containing vitamins A, D, E and omega-3 fatty acids, cod liver oil plays a vital role in human health. It assists in lowering cholesterol, reducing inflammation, enhancing memory, improving thyroid function, reducing asthma, improving glucose response, increasing cardiovascular health and benefiting intestinal disorders such as Crohn's disease, irritable bowel syndrome and colitis.

Cod liver oil has also shown benefits for those suffering with hypertension. The vitamin D contained in cod liver oil assists in the absorption of calcium and magnesium, which are necessary components of good blood pressure health. Moreover, the omega-3 component helps lower cholesterol.

Omega-3 Fatty Acids—Fat is not necessarily a bad word. In fact, there is an entire family of fat that is beloved by healthcare professionals because it is healthy for you. These fats are not only healthy, they are essential for your body. They are known as omega, or the omega-3 fatty acids.

Omega-3s are the good-for-you unsaturated fatty acids comprised of the polyunsaturated trio of a-linolenic acid (ALA), eicosapentaenoic acid (EPA) and docosahexaenoic acid (DHA). EPA and DHA have been awarded "qualified health claim" status by the Food and Drug Administration.

In the 1970s, researchers studied the diets of the Eskimos of Greenland and it was discovered that two of the three types of omegas (EPA and DHA) were essential to heart health. These fatty acids were ingested in large doses via the Eskimos' seafood-rich diet. Moreover, they showed almost no cardiovascular disease as these omega-3 fatty acids naturally reduce triglycerides and arterial plaque while reducing heart rate and maintaining healthy blood pressure.

Sources of omega-3 fatty acids include ocean-raised salmon, herring and mackerel, cod liver oil, olive oil, borage oil and flaxseed oil. Try making these a part of every meal and see how their benefits assist your natural blood pressure lowering program.

Magnesium—A 2012 meta-analysis published in the *European Journal of Clinical Nutrition*,[35] assessed the blood pressure lowering effectiveness of magnesium. In the studies they analyzed, the mean daily supplementation dose was 410 mg. They found a "small but clinically significant" blood pressure reduction.

CHINESE HERBAL PATENT MEDICINES

Chinese herbs are a main feature of traditional Chinese medicine. There are many ways to take Chinese herbals. These include in raw and cooked forms, as powders, in liquids and pills. Perhaps the most common way of taking Chinese herbs in the West is in the form known as the Patent Herbal Formulas. These are prepackaged herbal formulas that have been found effective for specific syndromes. They are bottles of small, BB-like pills that are coated in licorice and taken three per day, on average. Below are four patent formulas used in the treatment of hypertension.

Yang Yin Jiang Ya Wan—This formula contains anti- hypertensive, sedative and calmative properties. Designed specifically for hypertension, this formula contains several herbs with well-documented antihypertensive actions. The formula is best for treating high blood pressure in those who are also experiencing the following symptoms: Headache, dizziness, tinnitus, transient ischemic attacks, anger outbursts and sore eyes.

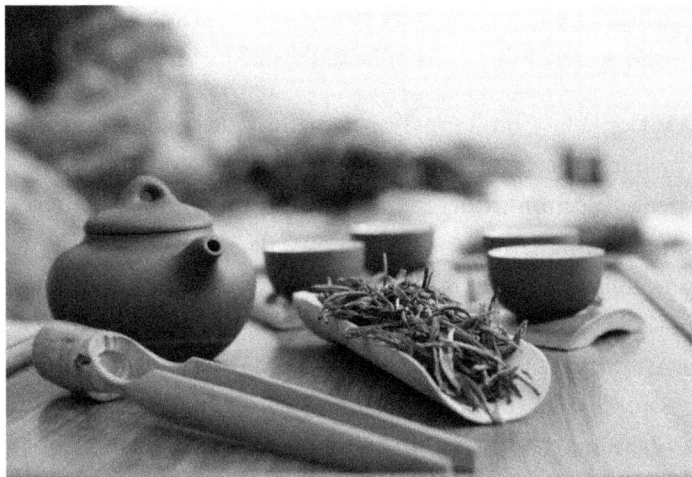

As Yang Yin Jiang Ya Wan is a formula and not a single herb, it consists of the following: Polygonatum multiflorum (he shou wu), cassia tora (jue ming zi, cassia seed), paeonia lactiflora (bai shao, white peony), poria cocos (fu ling, hoelen), eucommia ulmoides (du zhong, eucommia), alimsa orientale (ze xia, alisma), achyranthes bidentata (niu xi, achyranthes), bedendrobium nobile (shi hu, dendrobium), uncaria rhynchophylla (gout eng, gambir) and extracts equivalent to dry: Zea mays (yu mi xu, corn silk), poly-gonatum sibirica (yuan zhi, polygala) and chrysanthemum sinesis (ju hua, chrysanthemum flower).

Tian Ma Gou Teng Wan—This formula contains antihypertensive, sedative and calmative properties. This formula is best for treating high blood pressure in those who are also experiencing the symptoms of headaches on the sides or top of the head, neck and shoulder stiffness, dizziness, vertigo, facial flushing, irritability, insomnia and visual disturbances.

As Tian Ma Gou Teng Wan is a formula and not a single herb, it consists of the following: Viscum coloratum (sang ji sheng, vaecium), calcium sulfate (substitute for conch shell, shi jue ming), uncaria rhynchophylla (gout eng, gambir), polygonatum multiflorum (ye jiao teng, polygonatum stem), poria cocos (fu ling, hoelen), achyranthes bidentata (niu xi, achyranthes), leonurus sibirica (yi mu becoa, motherwort), gastrodia elata (tian ma, gastrodia), gardenia florida (shan zhi zi, gardenia) and eucommia ulmoides (du zhong, eucommia).

Tian Ma Wan—This formula contains antihypertensive, sedative and calmative properties. This formula is best for treating mild cases of high blood pressure in those who are also experiencing the symptoms of stiffness in the neck and shoulder.

As Tian Ma Wan is a formula and not a single herb, it consists of the following: Rehmannia glutinosa (sheng di, raw rehmannia), angelica polymorpha (dang gui, Chinese angelica), notopterygium incisum (qiang huo, notopterygium), eucommia ulmoides (du zhong, eucommia), gastrodia elata (tian ma, gastrodia), achyranthes bidentata (niu xi, achyranthes), Scrophularia ningpoensis (xuan shen, Scrophularia), dioscorea hypoglauca (bei xie, fish poison yam), angelica pubescens (du huo) and cyperus rotundus (xiang fu, cyperus).

Zhen Gan Xi Feng Wan—This formula contains antihypertensive, sedative and calmative properties. This formula is best for treating high blood pressure in those who are also experiencing symptoms of dizziness and vertigo, temporal and vertical headache, visual disturbances, tinnitus, facial flushing, tremors, disturbances of consciousness and hypertension.

PLEASE NOTE:

When taking supplements of any kind, it is best to discuss them with your doctor to research for reported contraindication with medication you may be taking. Moreover, it is best to get a solid recommendation from a healthcare professional and to only take the amount prescribed on the product packaging.

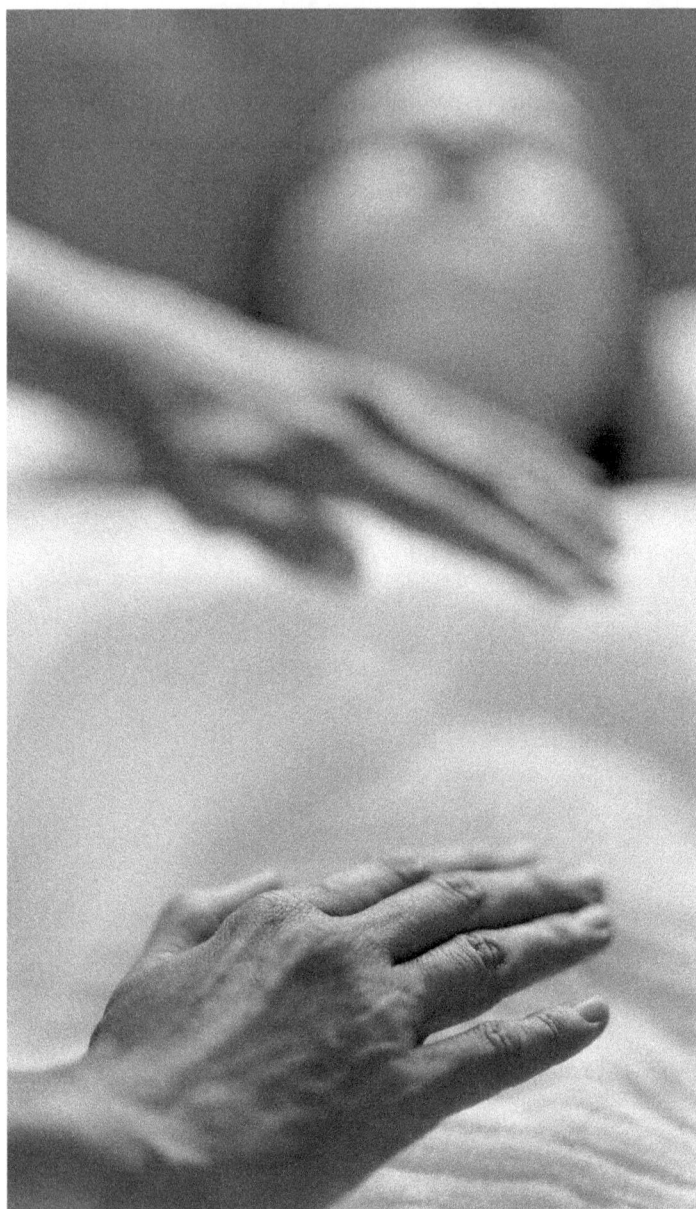

CHAPTER 7

Energy Medicine for Lowering Blood Pressure

Everything in the Universe is made up of energy and is vibrating at specific frequencies. Quantum physics has proven this to be fact. Human beings are essentially physical bodies constructed of various frequencies of energetic vibration. The quality of these vibrations can be controlled by our thoughts and are represented in every organ, system and fluid in our body. Sickness, therefore, equates to low- or poor-quality energetic vibrations in each of our cells.

All aspects of health and wellbeing—including hypertension—are tied to energetic frequencies. You must change your energetic frequency to feel better and live better. When you can do this, stress reduces, blood pressure normalizes and disorders such as overeating, drinking and smoking become a thing of the past.

THE ENERGY BODY

Traditional cultures around the world built their healing models on correcting energetic imbalances in the body.

Indeed, the role of Shamans in Siberia, Alaska and South-east Asia was to eradicate "bad spirits" (i.e., negative energy) from the body to restore physical or mental health in those suffering. The entire pantheon of Chinese and Indian healing practices was built on the premise of energy systems and pathways in the body that, when blocked, cause pain and disease. Clearing these channels or centers of blocked energy (e.g., toxins, spasms) is what restores health to the ill and offers relief to the pain sufferer.

Perhaps the most common term used to talk about human energy, is aura. This is a general term used to describe the color, mood or quality of five overlapping energy layers. These layers of energy (or "energy bodies") refer to the spiritual, mental, emotional, etherical and physical energies that make up humans.

Energy is developed, stored and moved in the body through the adrenals, the organs, chakra centers and meridian pathways. There is a saying in traditional Chinese medicine that tells why we experience pain: "Where there is energy blockage, there is illness. Where energy moves freely, there is no illness."

The key to pain relief and lasting health, then, is to open the energy channels, always raise your vibration frequency and keep your energy moving. There are several alternative therapies whose primary function is focused on just that. Let's look at a few here.

ACUPUNCTURE: ENERGETIC NEEDLE THERAPY

All Chinese body-healing practices are based on the idea that energy flows through the body in channels called meridians. These transport energy and life essence from organ to organ. Again, where there is slow energy or blockage, there is felt pain and soon disease.

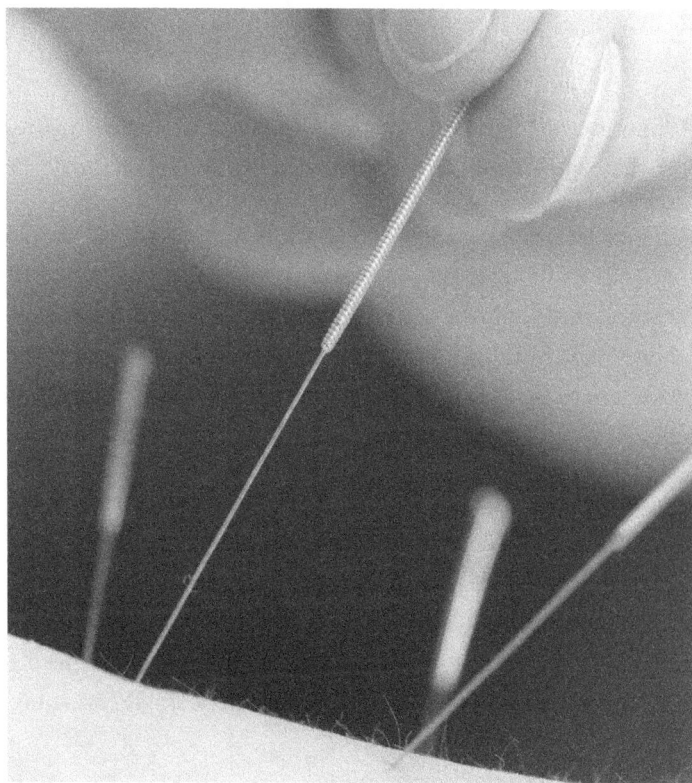

Acupuncture, one of the traditional Chinese medicine (TCM) modalities, is an ancient system of medicine in which fine needles are used by licensed practitioners to pierce the skin on specific points to a depth of a few millimeters. They are withdrawn after a period of about 28 minutes. The needles can be likened to an antenna, which draws in bioelectric energy into a very small port on the body, which then regulates the functions of the meridian system.

Using a correct "prescription" of points, the practitioner can in effect change the energy in a patient by opening their channels to help their energy move more freely. Again, when energy moves freely there is no disease.

Acupuncture is widely practiced today and worth looking into. It has been around for 5,000 years… not too shabby!

Atherosclerosis ("clogged arteries") is the result of plaque build-up in the arteries. Plaque is a substance comprised of fat, cholesterol, fibrin, calcium, cellular waste and other substances that build up along the arterial walls narrowing the space where oxygen-rich blood flows. If a blood clot forms as a result, it can break loose and cause heart attack or stroke.

In a three-way study, a specific form of acupuncture known as "threading," beat regular acupuncture and the statin drug Simvastatin (aka Zocor) in improving cardiovascular health. In acupuncture, a needle is normally inserted into a single acupoint. However, in the threading method, a single needle is threaded in a way to join two points with a single insertion.

STUDY: Acupuncture Lowers Blood Pressure

A trial published in the *Anhui Journal of Traditional Chinese Medicine*,[36] saw 216 patients with a diagnosis of primary hypertension were randomized into three active treatment groups: Ear acupuncture (N=72); corporal acupuncture (N=72); and a combination of ear and corporal acupuncture (N=72). Each group received a 20-minute treatment once a day for 10 days.

A significant effective response was defined as either the diastolic pressure returning to the normal range and the reduction was >10 mm/Hg, or the diastolic pressure reduction was greater than 20 mm/Hg even if the reduction did not return to the normal range.

All three groups showed a statistically significant reduction of blood pressure. In the combination ear and corporal acupuncture group, a significant effective response was observed in 43 out of 72 patients with a total response rate of 86.1%.

REIKI: A LAYING-ON OF HANDS

Reiki is a Japanese energy technique for reducing stress and inducing relaxation to help promote the free flow of energy in the body. To be most effective, Reiki requires the "laying on of hands" of a practitioner for its benefits to be gained.

Reiki practitioners place their hands-on patients in various configurations that are modeled on ancient Tibetan and Chinese powerful healing symbols. It is believed that re-creating these symbols on the body will allow "God's energy" to flow from the universe, through the practitioner and into the patient. This energy, which is vibrating at a high frequency, will lift the low energy of the sufferer to relieve pain and illness.

Reiki has become a popular healing modality among nurses in hospitals. The patient does not have to be awake for them to administer a few minutes of healing touch.

•••••

Hypertension is the result of excess energy in the blood pushing against the arterial walls. The above-mentioned energy medicine therapies are just a handful of those that can bring relief by correcting energetic imbalances in the body. They are based on thousands of years of trial-and-error application and have an amazing track record of success.

References Cited

Introduction

1. Centers for Disease Control and Prevention (CDCP). (2020). "Facts About Hypertension." https://www.cdc.gov/bloodpressure/facts.htm

2. American Heart Association. (2014). "Heart Disease and Stroke Statistics – At-a-Glance." https://www.heart.org/idc/groups/ahamah-public/@wcm/@sop/@smd/documents/downloadable/ucm_470704.pdf

3. Centers for Disease Control and Prevention (CDCP). (2017). "Hypertension." https://www.cdc.gov/nchs/fastats/hypertension.htm

Chapter 1: Hypertension and Its Risk Factors

4. WebMD (2020). "Hypertension/High Blood Pressure Health Center." http://www.webmd.com/hypertension-high-blood-pressure/default.htm

5. FamilyDoctor.org. (2018). "Heart Disease: Assessing Your Risk." https://familydoctor.org/heart-disease-assessing-your-risk/

6. Lloyd-Jones D. (2009). "Heart disease and Stroke Statistics—2009 Update." *Circulation*, 119 (3): 480-6.

7. Barsky AK. (2005). "Psychiatric and Behavioral Aspects of Cardiovascular Disease." In: Zipes, Libby, Bonow, Braunwald (Eds.). *Braunwald's Heart Disease: A Textbook of Cardiovascular Medicine. 7th ed.*, Philadelphia, Pa: WB Saunders: 2129-2144.

8. Merck Research Laboratories. *The Merck Manual of Diagnosis and Therapy. 18th ed.* Whitehouse Station, NJ. Merck & Co., Inc., 2006.

Chapter 2: Stress and Hypertension

9. WebMD. (2019). "Heart Disease and Stress: What's the Link?" http://www.webmd.com/hypertension-high-blood-pressure/guide/hypertension-easing-stress

10. Psychology Wiki. (nd). "Sleep Deprivation." https://psychology.wikia.org/wiki/Sleep_deprivation

11. King AC, Pruitt LA, Woo S, et al. (2008). "Effects of moderate-intensity exercise on polysomnographic and subjective sleep quality in older adults with mild to moderate sleep complaints." J Gerontol A Biol Sci Med Sci., 63 (9): 997-1004.

Chapter 3: Mind-Body Practices for Hypertension

12. Dwoskin D. (2007). The Sedona Method™. Arizona: The Sedona Press.

13. Chandratreya S. (nd). "Hypertension & Yoga." https://www.yogapoint.com/therapy/hypertension_yoga.htm

14. Harvard. (2011). "Eight weeks to a better brain." https://news.harvard.edu/gazette/story/2011/01/eight-weeks-to-a-better-brain/

15. Steinhubl SR, Wineinger NE, Patel S, et al. (2015). "Cardiovascular and Nervous System Changes During Meditation." https://www.frontiersin.org/articles/10.3389/fnhum.2015.00145/full

16. Lee MS, Lee MS, Choi ES, Chung HT. (2003). "Effects of Qigong on Blood Pressure, Blood Pressure Determinants and Ventilatory Function in Middle-Aged Patients with Essential Hypertension." *Am J Chin Med.,* 31(3): 489-97. https://www.ncbi.nlm.nih.gov/pubmed/12943180

17. Medical News Today. (2018). "Can Yoga Reduce Blood Pressure?" https://www.medicalnewstoday.com/articles/260699

Chapter 4: Exercise and Hypertension

18. Mayo Clinic. (2019). "Exercise: A Drug-Free Approach to Lowering High Blood Pressure." https://www.mayoclinic.org/diseases-conditions/high-blood-pressure/in-depth/high-blood-pressure/art-20045206

19. Aizer A, Gaziano JM, Cook NR, et al. (2009). "Relation of Vigorous Exercise to Risk of Atrial Fibrillation." Am J Cardiol., 103 (11): 1572–1577. https://www.ncbi.nlm.nih.gov/pmc/articles/PMC2687527/

20. Karjalainen, Jouko, et al. (1998). "Lone Atrial Fibrillation in Vigorously Exercising Middle Aged Men: Case-Control Study." *British Medical Journal*, 316: 1784-85.

21. Siegel AJ, Stec JJ, et al. (2001). "Effect of marathon running on inflammatory and hemostatic markers." https://www.ajconline.org/article/S0002-9149(01)01909-9/fulltext

22. Wang XJ & Moffett JPC. (1994). *Traditional Chinese Therapeutic Exercises–Standing Pole.* Foreign Languages Press: Beijing, China.

23. Agatston A. (2003). *The South Beach Diet: The Delicious, Doctor-Designed, Foolproof Plan for Fast and Healthy Weight Loss.* Random House.

24. WebMD. (2007). "A Little Walking Cuts Blood Pressure." https://www.webmd.com/hypertension-high-blood-pressure/news/20070815/a-little-walking-cuts-blood-pressure

Chapter 5: Diet and Hypertension

25. Blaustein MP. (2017). "The Pump, the Exchanger, and the Holy Spirit: Origins and 40-Year Evolution of Ideas About the Ouabain-Na+ Pump Endocrine System." *American Journal of Physiology-Cell Physiology.* https://doi.org/10.1152/ajpcell.00196.2017

26. Di Nicolantonio JJ and Lucan SC. (2014). "The Wrong White Crystals: Not Salt but Sugar as Aetiological In Hypertension and Cardiometabolic Disease." *Open Heart.* https://openheart.bmj.com/content/1/1/e000167

27. Jalal DI and Smits G, et al. (2010). "Increased Fructose Associates with Elevated Blood Pressure." *J Am Soc Nephrol.,* 21(9). https://www.ncbi.nlm.nih.gov/pmc/articles/PMC3013529/

28. Mitchell D. (2010). "Cut Soft Drink Consumption, Reduce Blood Pressure." ExamHealth. http://www.emaxhealth.com/1275/cut-soft-drink-consumption-reduce-blood-pressure.html

29. Science Daily (2013). "Drinking Cup of Beetroot Juice Daily May Help Lower Blood Pressure." https://www.sciencedaily.com/releases/2013/04/130415172230.htm

30. Arturo Figueroa A, Sanchez-Gonzalez MA, et al. (2010). "Effects of Watermelon Supplementation on Aortic Blood Pressure and Wave Reflection in Individuals with Prehypertension: A Pilot Study." *American Journal of Hypertension.* https://academic.oup.com/ajh/article/24/1/40/2281929

31. Ried K and Fakler P. (2014). "Potential of Garlic (Allium Sativum) in Lowering High Blood Pressure: Mechanisms of Action and Clinical Relevance." *Integr Blood Press Control.,*7: 71–82.

32. Med Page Today. (2016). "Study: Aged Cheese Lowers Blood Pressure: Small Randomized Trial Suggests Effect of Grana Padano on par with Antihypertensives." https://www.medpagetoday.com/meetingcoverage/ash/57924

33. Akilen R, Pimlott Z, et al. (2013). "Effect of Short-Term Administration of Cinnamon on Blood Pressure in Patients with Prediabetes and Type 2 Diabetes." *Nutrition,* 29 (10): 1192-1196. https://www.sciencedirect.com/science/article/abs/pii/S0899900713001913

34. Yang Q, Liu T, Kuklina EV, et al. (2011). "Sodium and Potassium Intake and Mortality Among US Adults: Prospective Data from the Third National Health and Nutrition Examination Survey." *Arch Intern Med., 171* (13): 1183-1191. https://jamanetwork.com/journals/jamainternalmedicine/fullarticle/1106080?resultClick=1

Chapter 6: Natural Supplements and Herbal Remedies

35. Kass L, Weekes J, Carpenter L, et al. (2012). "Effect of Magnesium Supplementation on Blood Pressure: A Meta-Analysis." *Eur J Clin Nutr., 66* (4): 411-418. https://www.ncbi.nlm.nih.gov/pubmed/22318649

Chapter 7: Energy Medicine for Lowering Blood Pressure

36. Lin X, Xing X. (1999). "Effects of Combination of Ear Acupuncture and Corporal Acupuncture on Lowering Blood Pressure." *Anhui Clinical Journal of Traditional Chinese Medicine*, 11 (2): 81.

About the Author

MARK WILEY, OMD, PhD, MS
Self-Directed Wellness Advocate

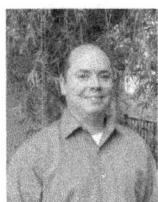

Mark has traveled extensively throughout the United States, Europe, the Philippines, Malaysia, Singapore, Taiwan, Hong Kong and Japan to research and master the world's alternative healing practices; from the oldest to the most modern. His interest in natural health practices was not just a mere curiosity; he was looking for long-lasting relief from the debilitating migraines and chronic pain that plagued him for most of his life. The combination of always being in pain and as a rebound of taking medications, he also developed high blood pressure later in life.

In search of a cure, when all else failed, Mark sought treatments from chiropractors, physical therapists, hypnotists, acupuncturists, herbalists, bonesetters, qigong masters, yoga masters, traditional Chinese doctors, faith healers and tribal shamans.

After decades of research, personal experience and education (Doctorates in both Oriental and Alternative Medicine and a

Masters in Healthcare Management), Mark saw the forest for the trees and developed an integrative self-directed wellness model he employed to rid himself of chronic headaches, body pain and hypertension. He helps others by writing on all aspects of wellness as an Advisor and Contributor to EasyHealthOptiions.com and The Healthy Back Institute. His articles and books continue to help hundreds-of-thousands of people around the globe achieve healthy, pain-free, balanced lives.

TAMBULI MEDIA

"EXCELLENCE IN MIND/BODY PUBLISHING"

Welcome to **Tambuli Media**, publisher of quality books and digital media on lifestyle, health, fitness, and traditional martial arts.

Our Vision is to see mind-body practices once again playing an integral role in the lives of people who pursue a journey of personal development to improve their lives and inspire others.

Our Mission is to partner with the highest caliber subject-matter experts to bring you quality content that is in-depth, professional, actionable and comprehensive in nature. We welcome you to join our Tambuli Family and to spend time on our site reading articles, watching videos, downloading content, and ordering products. Join one or more of our Email Lists to stay in touch and receive "Members Only" content, invitations to private webinars, and discount codes on new releases and bundled merchandise.

www.tambulimedia.com